Clinical
Challenges

Clinical
Challenges

Edited by

Judy Lumby and Debbie Picone

assisted by
Belinda Chaplin and Julienne Onley

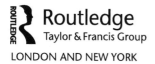

Routledge
Taylor & Francis Group

LONDON AND NEW YORK

First published 2000 by Allen & Unwin

Published 2020 by Routledge
2 Park Square, Milton Park, Abingdon, Oxon OX14 4RN
605 Third Avenue, New York, NY 10017

Routledge is an imprint of the Taylor & Francis Group, an informa business

National Library of Australia
Cataloguing-in-Publication entry:

Clinical challenges.

Includes index.
ISBN 1 86448 999 5.

1. Nursing. 2. Nursing—Practice. 3. Nursing—Social aspects.
I. Lumby, Judy. II. Picone, Debbie. (Series: Focus on nursing).

610.73

Set in 10/12pt Goudy by DOCUPRO, Sydney

ISBN-13: 9781864489996 (pbk)

Contents

Contributors   vii
Preface   ix

PART I   NURSING PRACTICE

1 MANAGING PAIN   3
   Isobel Taylor & Shirley Anne Wilson
   Commentary: Michael Cousins

2 MANAGING WOUNDS   24
   Keryln Carville
   Commentary: Tal Ellis

3 NURSE PRACTITIONERS   40
   Amanda Adrian & Jane O'Connell

4 THE NSW NURSE PRACTITIONER PROJECT   53
   Amanda Adrian & Jane O'Connell
   Commentary: Chris Murphy

PART II   INFLUENCE ON PRACTICE

5 SUICIDE   73
   Pierre Baume
   Commentary: Jennifer Chipps & Beverley Raphael

6 DRUG USE   98
   Kate Dolan
   Commentary: Richard Matthews

7   AGEING   118
    John Stevens & Julienne Onley
    Commentary: Irene Stein

8   EXTENDING LIFE   140
    Mary Chiarella
    Commentary: Michael Walsh

PART III   HEALTH CARE DELIVERY

9   CLINICAL INFORMATION SYSTEMS   159
    Dianne Ayres & Lyn Perks
    Commentary: Jeffrey Soar

10 HEALTH CARE AS A MARKET PLACE   176
    Debbie Picone
    Commentary: Kim Walker

11 ALWAYS IN THE RED   195
    Kerry Russell
    Commentary: Belinda Chaplin

Index   219

Contributors

Amanda Adrian, RN, LLB(UNSW) , BA(UNE), FCN(NSW), FRCNA, Director, Private Health Care Branch, NSW Health Department

Dianne Ayres, RN, MInfoCommTech, BAdmin(Nurs), CM, MCN (NSW), Manager, Clinical Systems, NSW Health Department

Pierre J.M. Baume, RN, RPB, DipAppScN , BappScN, MHP, DCH, FRCNA, FANZCMHN, Senior Consultant and Coordinator, Suicide Research and Prevention, Central Sydney Area Health Service

Keryln Carville, RN, BSc(Nsg), STN Cert., Clinical Nurse Consultant (Stomal Therapy/Wound Management), Silver Chain Nursing Association, Perth

Belinda Chaplin, RN, BBus, CC Cert, MCN(NSW), Director of Corporate Services, Corrections Health Service, NSW

Mary Chiarella, RN, CM, DipNEd(Dist), LLB(Hons), Associate Professor, Faculty of Nursing, Midwifery and Health, University of Technology, Sydney

Jennifer Chipps, RN, RPN, BSc(Nurs)(Psych)(Hons), MPH, GradDipEd, GradDipAd, GradDipEpi, Epidemiologist, Centre for Mental Health, NSW Health Department

Michael Cousins, AM, MD, FRCA, FANZCA, Professor and Head, Department of Anaesthesia and Pain Management, University of Sydney, Royal North Shore Hospital, Sydney

Kate Dolan, PhD, Research Fellow, National Drug and Alcohol Research Centre, University of NSW

Tal Ellis, RN, DipAppSci, BN, Lecturer, School of Nursing, Division of Health Services, University of South Australia

Judy Lumby, RN, PhD, MHPEd, BA, FCN(NSW), FRCNA, Executive Director, NSW College of Nursing

Richard Matthews, MBBS, Director of Clinical Services, Corrections Health Service, NSW

Chris Murphy, RGN, BSc(Hons), Health Studies/Nurse Practitioner (RCN/IANP), Nurse Manager, Primary Care, Corrections Health Service, NSW

Jane O'Connell, RN, MN, MCN(NSW), Clinical Nurse Consultant, Emergency Department, Concord Repatriation General Hospital, NSW

Julienne Onley, RN, MSc(Mental Health), Cert. Geront. Nursing, FCN(NSW), Manager, Professional Services and Policy, NSW College of Nursing

Lyn Perks, RN, RPN, BScN, DipCSM, MBA, Manager, Information Services, Princess Alexandra Hospital and District Health Service, Brisbane

Debbie Picone, RN, BHA(NSW), FCN(NSW), Chief Executive Officer, Corrections Health Service, NSW

Beverley Raphael, AM, MBBS, MD, FRANZCP, FASSA, FRCPsych, Director, Mental Health Services, NSW Department of Health

Kerry Russell, RN, BAdmin(Nsg), MgtCert., MCN(NSW), Director of Nursing, Concord Repatriation General Hospital, NSW

Jeffrey Soar, BA(Hons), GradDipCommercialDataProcessing, GradDipEd, Med, PhD, General Manager, Information Technology, New Zealand Police

Irene Stein, RN, PhD, MA, BHS, GerontNursCert., DNE, BA, Professor, Gerontological Nursing Research and Practice Unit, Baptist Community Services and the University of Newcastle, NSW

John Stevens, RN, BA(Hons), PhD, MRCNA, MCN(NSW), Senior Lecturer, School of Nursing, Southern Cross University and St Vincent's Hospital, Lismore, NSW

Isobel Taylor, RN, RPN, MidCert, OrthoCert., DipTeach, MN, FCN(NSW), Lecturer, Department of Anaesthesia and Pain Management Centre, Royal North Shore Hospital, Sydney

Kim Walker, RN, PhD, BAppSc, MCN(NSW), Director, Professional Services, NSW College of Nursing

Michael Walsh, SThD, Ethics Consultant

Shirley Anne Wilson, RN, DNE, FCN(NSW), Education Consultant, NSW College of Nursing

Preface

This book is the first of a planned series which positions nursing and nurses within the health care system in Australia, hence the title of the series, 'Focus on Nursing'. This volume highlights the numerous roles nurses occupy across the system, roles which are vital for quality care. For this reason, nurses have much to say about the system itself yet are often overlooked or under-represented when it comes to making key decisions.

While the chapters in this volume focus on contemporary issues central to the roles of nurses, they also flag potential pressures in the health care system itself which require more global attention and planning. The authors are mainly nurses actively involved in the system, some in clinical work, some as educators and others as managers or executives. Subsequent volumes will involve nurses from other sectors such as universities, research, and specific clinical specialties. The series is written for an audience of undergraduate and graduate nursing students as well as for nurses across the health and higher education sectors. It also has value for others working in the health care system who wish to be appraised of the points of concern for nurses.

To add to the dimensions of each chapter we invited specific commentators to provide additional perspectives to those of the author/s. In most cases they were invited because of their known stance on the issue at hand which we expected to be at odds with that taken by the author/s—although this has not always turned out to be the case.

This first volume, *Clinical Challenges*, is divided into three parts, each addressing a specific topic area chosen for its currency and impact. Part I is made up of clinically focused chapters. Two of these address areas of nursing practice that are central to safe and effective patient care—pain and wound management.

Despite pharmacological breakthroughs and our current knowledge of the multi-dimensional nature of pain, it still remains poorly managed as evidenced in the chapter 'Managing pain' where we learn that in 1992, 'less than 50% of surgical patients reported having adequate pain management in the post-operative period'. Children, patients with cancer and the aged fare no better, with research reflecting an overall dismal recognition of a patient's pain by nurses and doctors. Given their close relationship with such patients, nurses have the potential to change this situation. Isobel Taylor and Shirley Anne Wilson, two expert nurses in this area, have provided a thorough critique of the literature and context which surrounds the management of pain placing it, as Professor Michael Cousins points out in his commentary, where it belongs as a 'multi-dimensional problem'.

The companion chapter, 'Managing wounds', addresses another essential practice area in which nurses play a central role. The plethora of wound care information and products makes this area a minefield for the unwary. This chapter offers a path through the literature and available pharmaceuticals by analysing current practices and evidence. The author has created a fascinating chapter out of what some might imagine to be a sterile subject. Keryln Carville's historical analysis provides the background to what has been a contentious area of clinical practice. The move to a multi-disciplinary approach is similar to that of managing pain, shifts which auger well for the future of clinical practice in which the patient's needs are paramount. Chapters 1 and 2 make an important contribution to the current literature and would be valuable inclusions in the reading list of any undergraduate or post-graduate nursing program.

Two chapters addressing the nurse practitioner have been placed in Part I because of the potential nurse practitioners have to enhance clinical practice not only in terms of safety and effectiveness but also in terms of access for patients in areas of under-servicing. The historic nature of the *Nurses' Amendment (Nurse Practitioners) Act 1998* (NSW) (introduced in September 1998 by Dr Andrew Refshauge, the then Minster for Health and Minister for Aboriginal Affairs), makes the topic an essential inclusion in a book that focuses on contemporary nursing issues. This Act enabled nurse practitioners to become a reality in the health care system in New South Wales after years of lobbying, planning and research. By the time this volume is launched, our first nurse practitioners will be in place in rural and remote areas around the state. Acknowledging the extended roles that many nurses adopt in communities where they provide the primary care is a major stepping stone for nursing and for the communities in which these nurses work and live. Placing such roles within a recognised social, professional and legislative framework not only validates those who have been left to manage unsupported by the system but it also ensures that communities are cared for by an appropriately skilled, sensitive and well educated practitioner, whoever that may be.

Chapters 3 and 4 have been included because of their different foci. Chapter 3 is more global in terms of tracing the history and the debates surrounding what has been an extremely contentious issue within the health care system. Like all shifts that challenge the status quo of disciplinary boundaries, the move to establish nurse practitioner positions created its own momentum in terms of claims, misinformation and sensationalism. Rural communities were warned that the appointment of nurse practitioners would herald a range of disadvantages for them, including the withdrawal of medical services and poorer access to services in general. Such claims are unfounded and often mischievous. Indeed, nurse practitioners will provide increased services, usually in conjunction with a general practitioner where this is available. Nurse practitioners are not about taking over from doctors, but about providing a safe, effective service where a need is identified. This may be in an area where presently no doctor works or where a nurse practitioner can support and enhance medical practice.

Chapter 4 describes the project itself with its various stages. This provides an excellent example of the way in which an idea became a reality through strategic lobbying, careful planning and, most importantly, a united front professionally. Amanda Adrian and Jane O'Connell carefully highlight the critical issues arising from the research project in which they were both involved, as well as the Act itself which mandated further legislative amendments prior to the appointment of nurse practitioners. Presently, implementation of the various stages and amendments is proceeding smoothly and there is a palpable anticipation within the profession as we move closer to the first authorisation and appointment. This will be, in the words of the authors, the ultimate 'testament to the tenacity of many clinging to a vision based on the recognition of the health care needs of different populations'.

Part II addresses the effects on practice as we face an epidemic of social illnesses such as suicide and drug dependence. It is something of a paradox that at a time when medical science is making major breakthroughs in saving and extending lives we seem helpless in the face of rising rates of suicide and drug dependence, particularly in our youth. How we care for the health of our increasingly ageing population is also addressed here. It is a major social concern at a time when governments are reducing funding to aged people requiring care, those with mental and developmental disabilities and those needing social support. Compounding the devastating outcomes of these reductions has been the political rhetoric claiming that such strategies are to reduce society's dependence on handouts—rhetoric which reflects an outmoded paternalism, reactionary fiscal planning and detachment from the 'real' issues. The final chapter of Part II addresses one such real issue—the extension of life through medical intervention. This chapter juxtaposes the biological life with that of the biographical life through a critique of legal cases questioning the valuing of an individual life. As Mary Chiarella points out 'advances in science do not answer the questions about the value of the lives that have been extended'. For this reason it could be said that such a chapter does not belong in a book addressing health care, but as Dr Michael Walsh, the commentator, points out: 'nurses are involved in the continuing care of these patients and attempts to resuscitate, and are often in the best position to know the wishes of the patients'.

Nurses, by virtue of their role in the close and continuous care of patients, are privileged to hear the stories of people coping in times of illness, feeling vulnerable and at the mercy of the system. Such stories reveal that the health of a society is more than mortality rates and numbers of surgical interventions and more than clever science. It is about how we support those in our society who are unable to care for themselves so that we have a society in which the quality of life is at least reasonable for as many as possible. This means facing the difficult decisions about redistribution of funding, about what constitutes good health and a healthy society, about who should make the decisions and about whose interests should be served in a health care system. The issues raised in this section are by no means all encompassing of our major social ills and make no claims to be so. They are merely those that claim the attention of nurses today as they work towards addressing how to ensure better outcomes both for individuals and for society. But they can only do this if they are supported by a system with similar values and priorities.

Part III is devoted to health care delivery issues that may not necessarily be prescribed or managed by nurses but which have a major impact on how effectively nurses can carry out their roles. Chapter 9 concerns information systems as they have been and are developing in health care networks. Chapters 10 and 11 address structural issues, including the funding of the system in general and nursing in particular. While more descriptive in their format, the chapters in Part III provide essential information for nurses wherever they work in the system. This is the information that assists nurses to negotiate their way around what is a very complex and compartmentalised system, but one which they need to understand if they are to survive and thrive.

Clinical information systems are a relatively new field in our public health care system. Nurses and doctors have historically written patient notes, prescriptions and referrals by hand and in most places this tradition continues. However, there has been an increasing recognition of the lack of data available to those wishing to evaluate how well we are doing in health. What are the health gains of our society? What are we getting in return for the large amounts we are spending on health care? What trends can we identify? And for nursing, how can we show that we make a difference to the health outcomes of our patients? Unfortunately all these questions are difficult to answer with any accuracy because of the dearth of effective health care information systems in this country. As a result, our data tend to be intermittent and not predictive in terms of trends. So, while we have snap shots of clinical data, they are relatively useless in terms of future planning. This is about to change.

Dianne Ayres and Lyn Perks in their chapter, 'Clinical information systems', reinforce the vital role played by information in such a complex business as health. They claim that information technology is 'the enabler in integrating information across multiple care settings, reducing duplication and errors of omission, transcription and interpretation and providing timely information in the right location'. Effective information systems would go some way to overcoming the continuity of care problems identified by Debbie Picone in Chapter 10.

The infiltration of business strategies and rhetoric into the health care system has not gone unnoticed and indeed has received much criticism. Kim Walker's commentary on Chapter 10 engages with this critique providing another perspective to that provided by the author who situates herself as a senior health executive with 25 years clinical experience. Her contribution outlines the way in which our health care system is structured and funded and the many pressures currently influencing it. It also engages with some future predictions requiring strategic planning and management if we are to ensure a society that cares effectively and equitably for health care needs across sectors, cultures and geographical areas. Nurses at all clinical levels need to understand the issues outlined in 'Health care as a market place' if they are to be effective advocates for patients.

The final chapter in Part III addresses two major management problems for nurses at different levels of the system—rostering and resource management. Kerry Russell, a Director of Nursing, outlines an innovative model of rostering that recognises the need for a more family-friendly, flexible workplace in a system which is notoriously inflexible. At a time when nursing workforce issues are being debated at national level, when the critical shortage of nurses across all specialties is being addressed through recruitment and retention strategies, little is being done to address concerns of present staff about a workplace which is inflexible and unfriendly in terms of family life. This innovative rostering system is designed to overcome such barriers and therefore attract and retain staff.

This book represents the collective efforts of many, all working full time in their area of expertise. We acknowledge the willingness of authors and commentators to contribute to this volume in addition to their substantial work load. The assistant editors, Belinda Chaplin and Julienne Onley, also deserve acknowledgement for their hard work in managing the writers, formatting, editing and copying.

This is our first collaborative effort as editors. Each of our backgrounds contrasts with and complements the other. Somehow we managed to make our differences work effectively in terms of editing this book and in the process have both learned from the other. We hope that this book works for you and look forward to comments, feedback and suggestions for future volumes.

Judy Lumby & Debbie Picone
Sydney, 1999

PART I

Nursing practice

1 Managing pain

Isobel Taylor & Shirley Anne Wilson

INTRODUCTION

> Just as 'my pain' belongs in a unique way only to me, so I am utterly
> alone with it. I cannot share it. I have no doubt about the reality of
> the pain experience, but I cannot tell anybody what I experience.
> I surmise that others have 'their' pain, even though I cannot perceive
> what they mean when they tell me about it. I am certain about the
> existence of their pain only in the sense that I am certain of my
> compassion for them. And yet, the deeper my compassion, the deeper
> is my certitude about the other person's utter loneliness in relation to
> his experience (Illich 1976, p. 147).

Pain is among the most complex and at the same time the most
threatening of all the domains of ordinary human experience. The
quotation above highlights the very personal nature of the pain
experience and the bleak sense of loneliness when the experience
cannot be conveyed to another. However, in the presence of a compassionate and knowing other, this pain and loneliness can be
acknowledged and ameliorated. The compassionate acknowledgement
of pain and a resolve to ameliorate pain are primary responsibilities
of nurses towards patients in pain.

At the beginning of this century we have the knowledge and the
means to control pain as never before. Why then is there continuing
evidence that people are still suffering unacceptable levels of pain as
a result of surgery, trauma or disease? This chapter will examine the
ongoing factors impeding effective pain management and will discuss
the educational and institutional reforms that need to be initiated in
order to improve pain control.

The under-treatment of pain

A report commissioned by the Agency for Health Care and Policy and Research in 1992 found that less than 50% of surgical patients reported having adequate pain management in the post-operative period (AHCPR 1992). Studies undertaken in general surgical wards (Donovan, Dillon & McGuire 1987; Miaskowski 1993) and intensive care units (Puntillo & Weiss 1994; Puntillo & Wilkie 1991; Tittle & McMillan 1994) all showed that up to 75% of post-surgical patients reported moderate to severe pain which was inadequately managed. Despite advances in knowledge and technology these statistics are disappointingly similar to those reported by Marks and Sachar as long ago as 1973.

Research indicates that 71 to 83% of frail elderly living in aged care facilities experience severe pain, over one half of them on a daily basis (Ferrell, Ferrell & Osterwell 1990) while children often undergo painful procedures without adequate analgesic cover (Southall, Cronin & Hartmann 1993). Pain control in cancer, although improved since the advent of palliative care and the hospice movement, is sometimes not well managed in acute hospitals or general practice (Furstenberg et al. 1998).

Why do medical and nursing staff not recognise that their patients are in pain? If they do recognise it, why do they not act to control it? What is it that constrains them? Many studies, including those mentioned above, have sought to identify the reasons for the under treatment of pain. Most identify the reasons in terms of barriers to assessment and management. These are consistently identified as knowledge deficits, erroneous beliefs and attitudes of both health care professionals and patients towards pain and analgesics. Barriers relating to the health care and hospital systems are less frequently identified and yet the socio-political factors inherent in those systems may constitute a major impediment to effective pain management.

The nature of pain

Pain is a multi-dimensional phenomenon and a biopsychosocial construct. It needs acknowledgement as being moulded both by the person experiencing it and by the particular context within which it is experienced. Pain perception is a combination of physical, psychological and environmental factors; it is influenced by past experiences and learning, as well as culture.

To study pain and find the means to control it necessitates finding ways of describing it that are universal and contribute in a constructive way to pain discourse. The International Association for the Study of Pain (IASP), in a well recognised definition, states that: '. . . pain is an unpleasant sensory and emotional experience associated with actual or potential tissue damage, or described in terms of such damage . . .' (Merskey 1979). Notes accompanying this definition emphasise that pain is always subjective. Each individual learns the application of the word through experiences related to injury in early life. It is always an unpleasant and therefore emotional experience. Pain impacts on a person's psychosocial as well as physical functioning. In this way it is a complex experience not determined by tissue damage alone.

The subjective nature of the pain experience was emphasised by McCaffery over 30 years ago when she published this definition of pain: Pain is 'whatever the experiencing person says it is, existing whenever the experiencing person says it does' (McCaffery 1968, p. 95). McCaffery's definition and that of the IASP encompass the multi-dimensional nature of the pain experience. McCaffery's statement emphasises that the patient's self-report of pain is fundamental to the nursing assessment of pain. There is now extensive literature concerning the advances in knowledge related to pain physiology (Siddall & Cousins 1997). New knowledge has not only changed the definitions and classifications of pain but has significantly influenced pharmacological research and management. Clinicians need an understanding of the mechanisms of pain transmission and modulation if good clinical decisions are to be made regarding the control of pain.

BARRIERS RELATED TO PAIN ASSESSMENT

Scarry (1985) noted that while to feel pain is to have certainty, to hear about pain is to have doubt. The multi-dimensional nature of pain makes assessment of pain a complex issue. Patients are disadvantaged if they are managed by clinicians who operate from a biomedical model and whose education has emphasised objective signs as the gold standard for patient assessment. Lack of knowledge and insight will also affect the clinician's intention to assess the patient for pain, particularly if there is a concomitant lack of knowledge of the patient's culture (Walker, Tan & George 1995).

Within the biomedical framework, assessment of pain relies primarily on biological factors. This is a reductionist approach that assumes the pain problem results solely from neural and biochemical processes associated with pathology (Good et al. 1994). A prime example of this is seen when the timing and amount of post-operative analgesia is based solely on the type of operation performed. Assessing only the uni-dimensional intensity of pain ignores the cognitive, affective and social impact of surgery and hospitalisation. Relying on the patient's self-report of the nature and intensity of their pain should be a fundamental principle of pain assessment. The patient has a key role in successful management since only the patient knows where the pain is and how much it hurts. However, several factors, including the culture of the patient and nurse as well as the quality of the patient–nurse interaction, will influence the ability or willingness of the patient to express pain and the nurse to hear what is being said. Inadequate or erroneous knowledge about pain assessment is a major factor in poor pain control. If clinicians do not accept and act upon a patient's report of pain or fail to ask patients about pain, then the fundamental basis of pain assessment is compromised from the beginning. When patients' reports of pain are elicited but minimised or not even believed, then under treatment is the likely outcome.

One of the principles of pain management highlighted in the National Health and Medical Research Council (NH&MRC) guidelines under the heading 'Safe and effective analgesia' is frequent assessment and reassessment of pain intensity and meticulous documentation of pain assessment and efficacy of analgesia. It is necessary to distinguish between assessment and measurement of pain. Measurement requires quantification of one aspect of pain intensity and is uni-dimensional. Assessment encompasses the entire multi-dimensional pain experience and requires acknowledgement of the psychological and social impact of pain.

FACTORS RELATED TO MODELS OF CARE IN INSTITUTIONS

There is no evidence to support the notion that pain relief is prejudicial to diagnosis. Over a decade ago, a study of patients who presented to an emergency department with abdominal pain showed that there was no difference in accuracy of diagnosis or treatment outcome in those who were given analgesia before diagnosis compared to those who were not (Zoltie & Cust 1986).

Even when the education of nurses and doctors has inculcated the biopsychosocial approach, aspects of the socialisation that take place in the biomedical framework in which they work seems to disable numbers of them in dealing with pain and suffering. Good et al. (1994) argue that the biomedical framework restricts clinicians' humanity. It is possible that some clinicians can only prevent themselves from feeling overwhelmed or powerless in the face of pain and suffering by simply not acknowledging it or by denying accountability for it (Clements & Cummings 1991).

A sociological analysis of the problem of pain was published as far back as 1977 by Fagerhaugh and Strauss. It provided an enlightened perspective on the complexity of the pain experience in hospital. It was an extensive study comprising two years of observation in 20 different ward settings. The authors concluded that failure to adequately treat pain could be ascribed in part to the following factors:

- no one member of the team was actually accountable for relieving pain
- staff were caught up in recording physical signs, arranging and performing tests and procedures and documenting the drugs dispensed.

The observers in the study noted that nursing activities were not directly concerned with how the patient experienced and responded to pain and discomfort, while the organisational setting and interactive style of patient–staff encounters militated against effective pain management. The authors described the way in which some interactive processes (these were termed political acts) were used to compel patients to conform to the organisational needs of the ward, requiring them to tolerate significant pain in order to do this. Twenty years later, these statements have an all too familiar ring. In the climate of budget and staffing cuts, pain management still leaves much to be desired.

The literature is replete with studies that identify barriers to relieving patients' pain, including many factors related to clinicians, institutions and politics, as well as to patients and their families. One widely reported factor is the seemingly inadequate knowledge of doctors and nurses in relation to pain assessment and management (Francke et al. 1996; Graffam 1990; Zalon 1993) Another persistent and erroneous belief leading to under treatment of pain is based on fear of inducing addiction in patients. As long ago as 1980, Porter and Jick established that the incidence of addiction in patients given opiates for pain was extremely low and did not support the belief that addiction was a significant risk. Unfortunately some clinicians still adhere to this misconception. Patients with cancer and their relatives may fear that tolerance to the analgesia will develop and therefore they may want to 'hold off' until the pain becomes extremely bad. Again, this is a misconception shared by some clinicians.

Significant barriers exist within the treatment setting. These are partly related to nurse/doctor relationships and institutional constraints of funding for services. Some doctors seem to respond more readily to scientific or technological discourse about patients. Wicks (1999), in relating a conversation between a doctor and a nurse regarding a patient's suffering, observed that the conversation had no point at which the two could meet. Wicks postulated that the nurse was describing what was happening *for* the patient, while the doctor was relaying what was happening *to* the patient. If a nurse's skills and opinions are not valued by medical colleagues, then the doctor may not accept the nurse's reporting of the patient's pain, pain which may change over time. The nature of the doctor's contact with patients is more episodic and does not allow the observation over time that nurses maintain. A comprehensive picture of the patient's pain and responses to interventions will not be fully appreciated and could lead to under treatment if the doctor, who is the prescriber, is the sole arbiter of analgesic requirements. However, nurses are ideally placed to recognise and treat fear, anxiety and distress when interacting with patients, typically over an eight hour period. Anxiety reduction, for example, is known to be a factor in decreasing pain perception (Scott, Clum & Peoples 1983) and anxiety can be better recognised over longer contact time with a patient.

NURSING ISSUES IN PAIN MANAGEMENT

Procedural pain

Many patients are subjected to painful procedures in the course of treatment, often performed without appropriate analgesia. These procedures take place in many settings, the intensive care unit being one such environment. It is not hard to imagine the dread the patient feels in anticipation of the next approach by the nurse or doctor if analgesia is not given. After enduring intense procedural pain patients often report feeling victimised, violated or attacked (McCaffery & Pasero 1999). Before beginning a procedure, clinicians should discuss whether analgesics and sedatives might be needed. The decision to provide analgesia during a procedure should be based on the likelihood that it is going to produce pain. These discussions will be facilitated if standardised pain management protocols for particular procedures have been established in the unit. These protocols should include guidelines about the use of anxiolytics and sedatives as well as analgesics. In addition, the patient needs to understand what is about to happen and be aware of how the pain is to be managed. The patient's report of pain during the procedure is a reliable indicator of the intensity of the pain. If a conscious patient is unable to talk, an alternative signal should be established that can be used to alert the clinician if the pain is unacceptable.

In an unconscious patient observations reveal pathophysiological changes taking place in the nervous system in the absence of inadequate pain control. Although the patient cannot report the pain, changes in vital signs, muscular rigidity, groaning and grimacing are all reliable signs. Even in the absence of overt signs, the patient should be given the benefit of the doubt and receive analgesia before procedures that are known to be painful.

Acute post-operative pain

Acute pain teams are available in many hospitals. A key factor in this type of service is the use of technology to deliver analgesia, either intravenously or epidurally. Patient controlled analgesia (PCA) has been heralded as a major breakthrough in pain management but some audits of such services reveal that there is still a significant amount of unrelieved post-operative pain. An obvious advantage of PCA is that the patient has control over analgesic dosing. The machine responds instantly to a request from the patient (the patient presses a button) and delivers a set dose of analgesia. Overdose is guarded against by the lockout interval preventing dosing again until it is safe to do so. The patient's role in this type of pain management is as primary assessor of the pain. Not all post-operative patients have access to PCA machines since there are still insufficient available. Ironically, staff members may seem reluctant to administer the maximum allowed amount of prescribed analgesia to one patient while the patient in the next bed on a PCA machine is 'believed' by the machine and given pain relief on demand. An extremely valuable result of PCA technology is that it has highlighted the variability of pain levels among patients and the variable responses to opiates and other drugs. Despite these technological and pharmacological advances the problem of poor pain control persists. Perhaps these advances have added to the problem. It may be that some nurses and doctors abrogate their responsibility by relying solely on the machines and drugs to solve the pain problem and fail to adequately assess individuals' responses and to take appropriate action when pain is not adequately relieved. These issues are currently being addressed in the literature in Australia and the United Kingdom. Recent publication of an evidence-based approach to acute pain management (NH&MRC 1999; McQuay & Moore 1998) provides detailed recommendations for improved assessment and management of acute pain.

Neonatal pain

Despite advances in knowledge about pain in neonates some misconceptions have persisted leading to under treatment of pain. A major misconception is that neonates do not feel pain as much as adults or, if they do, they will not remember it and no harm will be done. It is now accepted on good evidence that the neurophysiological components required for pain perception are in place by 20 weeks gestation and are operational by pre-term delivery (Fitzgerald 1994). Non-painful stimuli such as bathing, recording vital signs and touch can be perceived as painful in the now altered physiological state of the neonate exposed to unrelieved pain (Fitzgerald, Millard & Macintosh 1989). The under treatment of acute pain puts neonates at risk of increased sensitivity to later painful events, for example, immunisation, or even of developing chronic pain syndromes (Taddio, Stevens & Craig 1997). The evidence for these altered states means that there is an ethico-legal imperative to adequately manage neonatal pain, quite apart from the humanitarian aspects of reducing suffering. Francke and Miaskowski (1997) published an extensive literature review of the available measurement tools including biological, physiological and biochemical parameters and concluded that, although blood assays for catecholamine levels may be a reliable measure, physiological and behavioural responses are cheaper and easier to obtain.

Pain in children

Pain management in children is now well documented with the more recent work focusing on pain assessment practices and nurses' decision making. Studies by Margolius, Hudson and Michel (1995) show that staff with the least amount of paediatric experience held the greatest number of misconceptions regarding pain management in children. Paediatric pain is more difficult to assess than in adults due to the complexities of cognitive development. It is therefore crucial that whatever tool is used it is appropriate to the cognitive development of the child being assessed. It is important that the parents are consulted about the child's responses regarding pain in the past as well as in the current situation.

Since there are so many assessment tools available there is a significant need for each clinical unit to have a protocol for each method. Staff education is vital to ensure reliable measurement and interpretation of scores.

Pain in the elderly

For many elderly people pain interferes with their activities of daily living and there is evidence to support the premise that they are vulnerable to inadequate pain management (Ferrell 1991). Attitudes of some clinicians, the community and the patients themselves reinforce the misconception that pain just has to be tolerated. However, assessment of pain in the elderly patient can be complex. Many elderly people consider pain as part of the ageing process or, in contrast, report feelings of loss and loneliness as physical pain. Caution about the use of analgesic and adjunctive drugs contribute to under treatment (Ferrell 1991). It is acknowledged that pain assessment can be hindered by altered sensory, affective and cognitive states. However, existing pain assessment tools can be used successfully as part of a comprehensive assessment (Ferrell et al. 1995). Visual analogue scales and faces rating scales can be used in some cognitively impaired patients provided that the nurse manages the environment in order to minimise distraction and engage the patient's attention. Speaking clearly and slowly and using appropriate language helps. Even if staff cannot elicit a patient report of pain, they cannot assume there is no pain. Common sense regarding behavioural cues such as facial expression, body movements, repetitive movements, yelling, striking out at staff and unwillingness to move should alert the nurse to the fact that there may be pain, particularly if the patient has a condition normally known to be painful or is being subjected to interventions that are usually considered to be painful. Reluctance to prescribe or administer analgesia in these circumstances is, in part, due to lack of knowledge of appropriate dosages for the elderly. A legitimate concern is that altered pharmacokinetics due to the ageing process may lead to an increased risk of toxicity and drug interactions.

For many elderly people pain diminishes their quality of life. They deserve access to the full range of treatment strategies available and should not be excluded from effective management because of their age or clinical complexity.

Chronic pain

Chronic non cancer pain is pain persisting beyond the usual time course of healing or associated with a chronic pathological process that causes ongoing or recurrent pain. It was previously thought that the pain needed to be present for three to six months before it could be classified as chronic. However, current practice guidelines consider that if it is left so long before treatment is initiated, then the result can be a sub-optimal outcome. Unlike acute pain, chronic pain is not accompanied by observable altered physiology, thus clinicians who rely on such alterations for confirmation of pain will be misled into doubting its existence, even in the face of a patient's report of pain. Post-herpetic neuralgia and phantom pain are just two examples of chronic neuropathic pain syndromes following nerve damage which can persist for a long time.

The chronic pain patient is particularly disadvantaged in the biomedical framework where the importance of diagnosis before treatment is no longer appropriate. For many chronic pain sufferers there is no diagnosis yet they can be helped to regain their lives despite the pain. Some patients are subjected to multiple costly investigations in the quest for a diagnosis and, in the absence of one, may find themselves relegated to the psychiatrist's couch.

CANCER PAIN AND SUFFERING

Patients with cancer may have multiple pain problems, including those due to tumour progression and related pathology. Nerve damage resulting in varying types of acute and chronic pain is particularly difficult to manage, while invasive diagnostic procedures and also surgery cause acute and ongoing pain. Treatment with chemotherapy and radiotherapy results in side effects that very often include pain; infection and reduced mobility are other factors that add to the pain experience. Moreover, emotions relating to actual or anticipated losses, grief, anger and fear of a painful death all exacerbate pain. Emotional pain may be unacknowledged by the patient, who may find it more bearable to somatise the suffering as physical pain. Clinicians may also find it easier to react to reports of physical pain rather than respond to messages of psychosocial suffering. The ability of the nurses who are caring for the patient to enter into a compassionate relationship with the patient is crucial to alleviate suffering. Just (1997, p. 59) offers a simple operational definition of compassion as: 'being with the patients in their suffering and not going away'.

This statement implies that there is a partnership between nurse and patient and a sense of undertaking a journey together. Just (1997) describes compassionate nurse counselling as developing the ability to keep the heart open to the patients and their stories no matter what happens. The open heart becomes the tool for 'being with' the patient. The emergence of palliative care in hospital and hospice settings has resulted in improved pain and symptom management for patients with cancer pain. The environment is one in which the focus is caring and symptom control rather than one where cure is the focus. On the other hand, when cancer patients are treated in settings where the biomedical model is the dominant framework they are at risk of experiencing unrelieved suffering.

EDUCATIONAL ISSUES AND PAIN

In response to a need for a more concerted approach to the study and treatment of pain a number of organisations were formed in the 1970s and 1980s. IASP published a core curriculum for professional education in pain. Practice guidelines have been published for cancer pain (AHCPR 1994), acute pain (AHCPR 1992) and by the NH&MRC in Australia (NH&MRC 1999). Yet these and other new concepts and knowledge have failed to improve the lot of many patients who still suffer preventable pain.

We believe the failure has arisen because the dominant framework within which many nurses and doctors practice is the biomedical model. Clinicians whose mindset is dominated by the biomedical model concentrate on neurophysiological aspects, both in assessment and treatment. In this way scientific medicine reduces the experience of pain to an elaborate broadcasting system of mechanistic signals. For some clinicians pain is simply a stimulus response that is a useful warning or clinical sign. The Cartesian split between mind and body is often cited as the basis for the dualism within the biomedical discourse about pain. It is somewhat unfair that Descartes is blamed for this state of affairs. The system he described for the first time in 1644 was indeed the simple stimulus–response nature of noxious input. In fact, this concept was a major advance for the time. Descartes envisaged a new and better world based on reason, a new era that signified an end to the ignorance and superstition that had dominated the discourse about pain in those times (Bendelow & Williams 1995).

Levin, Berry and Leiter (1998) attempted to summarise the studies to date related to investigation of practice and knowledge of palliative care physicians. The summary of the report emphasised the futility of traditional education to improve practice and noted that to effect change in behaviour, more is necessary than learning facts. Culture, experience, motivation, peer acceptance and initial socialisation to the practice setting all have some influence on behaviours. Is there a lack of role models in academic institutions as well as clinical practice? Does this account for improvement of knowledge with little change in practice? All clinicians and educators in health and health-related fields need to adopt an approach to pain as a quality issue and consider it an issue as fundamental as universal precautions against infection.

Education needs to be such that clinicians feel empowered to deliver care that is not only technically competent but, above all, humane. Lack of accountability for patients' pain is reflected in the results of a study in which 353 hospitalised patients were asked about their pain experience: 55% reported that no member of the health team had asked about pain and no documentation regarding pain was entered in the patient record (Donovan, Dillon & McGuire 1987). More recently, a study of 242 hospitalised patients revealed that no assessment of pain intensity was documented (Gu & Belgrade 1993).

Evidence-based practice and practice guidelines for pain management

As in most branches of medicine, pain management is being subjected to rigorous evaluation for evidence of efficacy and accuracy (McQuay & Moore 1998). In 1997 the NH&MRC commissioned a working party consisting of clinicians from all disciplines to produce clinical practice guidelines for the management of acute pain. These guidelines have now been published and are available on the NH&MRC web page (NH&MRC 1999). The acute pain guidelines have been written in a way that enables readers to judge the strength of the evidence on which the recommendations are based.

While there is a strong imperative in medicine to use evidence-based and quantitative research as a guide to practice it should be acknowledged that qualitative research designs provide a rich description of the relationship between clinicians' beliefs about pain and suffering and actual pain management. Similarly, insights into patient responses to pain and suffering uncovered by qualitative studies may help to provide the means to abolish many barriers to effective pain control (Warden, Carpenter & Brockopp 1998). In order that people with pain become beneficiaries of optimum pain relief there is a need for multi-disciplinary collaboration between clinicians and other health care providers. The foundation of this collaboration is education. Clinicians, patients, administrators and politicians need access to the new concepts of pain and its management in order to start realising this goal. No amount of empirical information about pain can help the clinician whose fundamental concepts and attitudes towards pain are outmoded. Pleas for appropriate funding and distribution of services for pain control will fall on deaf political and administrative ears unless it is demonstrated that poorly managed pain has economic and social costs society cannot afford.

Since nurses are involved in patient care around the clock, spending more time in contact with patients than other team members, it is a serious situation indeed if the nurse lacks the appropriate knowledge, skills and attitudes to assess pain. If a comprehensive picture of the patient's response to pain and interventions is to be transmitted to doctors and nursing colleagues, regular assessment of pain and treatment outcomes need to be documented as meticulously as other clinical data such as blood pressure, pulse and temperature. In the light of what is known about neural plasticity in reponse to noxious stimulation, it makes good sense to take steps to prevent or reduce pain occurring.

Nurses are well placed to influence patients' perceptions of pain. They can reduce anxiety by listening to patients' stories about previous encounters with pain and how they coped or how they did not cope. Explaining to surgical patients what to expect and how they will be helped is a prerequisite for reducing anxiety. Treating the operation as 'just routine' is likely to have the opposite effect to what is intended by such utterances. An operation or even a test, no matter how minor, is not routine to the person about to experience it. Pain assessment should begin at admission, establishing a pain history; questions related to previous painful episodes, their management and outcomes are as necessary as those questions used to elicit past medical history and fitness for anaesthesia.

Ethico-legal issues in pain management

There are ethico-legal implications for nurses and other clinicians for the recognition and treatment of pain. The code of ethics for nurses in Australia, developed in 1993 under the auspices of the Australian Nursing Council (ANC), includes the following explanatory note under its first value statement: 'Respect for individual needs, beliefs and values includes culturally sensitive care, and the provision of as much comfort, dignity, privacy and alleviation of pain and anxiety as possible' (ANC 1993).

In order to meet ethical standards of nursing care in relation to pain, nurses need to know and understand all of the possibilities now available for its management. The recent publication of guidelines for practice highlights accountability for pain management and that it becomes a liability issue. Health care professionals' attitudes towards pain should be subjected to critical examination in the light of new research and clinical realities. It is only as our concept of pain approximates the daily complexity of community and hospital life that we can comprehend pain and suffering sufficiently to control and relieve it.

THE MISUSE OF PLACEBOS IN PAIN MANAGEMENT

The placebo phenomenon is much misunderstood and consequently misused. Many clinicians believe, wrongly, that individuals who experience pain relief when given an inactive substitute for analgesia are not in real pain and are thus deceiving the staff. The misuse of placebos in pain management is considered by many nurses to be unethical. Elderly people in residential care are at risk of being prescribed placebos as analgesia because there is a lot of uncertainty about prescribing analgesics in this age group. The only place for placebo use is in controlled clinical trials.

The Oncology Nursing Society of America has issued a position statement on the use of placebos for pain management, summarised as follows: placebos should not be used to assess or manage cancer pain, to determine if pain is 'real', or to diagnose psychological problems such as anxiety associated with pain. Nurses should not administer placebos in these circumstances, even if there is a medical practitioner's order to do so. The American Society of Pain Management Nurses' position statement opposes the use of placebos for the treatment of pain in any patient (McCaffery & Pasero 1999).

It is a basic human right to expect relief of pain. Some statements have emerged which recognise this. A cancer care group in the United States published a bill of rights to encourage patients, their families and care givers to learn the facts about pain and its treatment. There are three statements that, if adopted universally, would reform the practice of pain management. These are:

- I have a right to have my reports of pain accepted and acted upon by health care professionals.
- I have the right to have my pain controlled, no matter what its cause or how severe it may be.
- I have the right to be treated with respect at all times. When

I need medication for pain, I should not be treated like a drug abuser.

Patients are often told they must expect to have pain and so are encouraged (or coerced) not to request analgesia until the pain is moderately severe for fear of being labelled as 'wimps'. This especially applies to young males (Cohen 1980; McInnes 1976).

Cautionary tales have appeared in the literature describing court actions initiated by patients and relatives because of instances of inadequate pain relief. Langslow (1992) cites a South Australian case in 1980 where an orthopaedic patient's pain was ignored by his surgeon with disastrous consequences for the patient. The surgeon and physiotherapists involved in this case had labelled the patient as having a low pain threshold common to his nationality (Italian) and as being given to histrionics. Thereafter they simply disregarded his reports of pain. The judge concluded that this failure to listen to the patient's complaints of pain amounted to negligence and awarded $77 690 to the plaintiff (Langslow 1992).

CONCLUSION

Despite better drugs, new technology and the presence of pain management teams, pain management is still sub-optimal. The reductionist and hierarchical approach still employed by many clinicians is inadequate and must be replaced by a wholistic multi-disciplinary team approach including psychosocial, cultural and patient-specific elements. Features of effective teams are cooperative management and mentoring of all members of the care team. Multi-disciplinary pain centres provide a rich environment for collaborative research, teaching and clinical practice. Comprehensive guidelines and standards have been published. The challenge for organisations and all of the members of the care team is to incorporate these standards into their philosophy and clinical practice.

REFERENCES

AHCPR (1992) *Clinical Practice Guidelines: Acute Pain Management: Operative or Medical Procedures of Trauma*, Rockville, MD: AHCPR pub. no. 92–0032.
AHCPR (1994) *Current Clinical Practice Guidelines: Management of Cancer Pain*, Rockville, MD: AHCPR pub. no. 94–592.
ANC (1993) *Code of Ethics for Nurses in Australia*, Canberra: Australian Nursing Council.

Baker, C.M. and Wong, D.L. (1987) 'Quest: A process of pain assessment in children', *Orthopaedic Nursing*, vol. 6, no. 11, pp. 11–22.

Bendelow, G.A. and Williams, S.J. (1995) 'Transcending the dualisms: Towards a sociology of pain' *Sociology of Health and Illness*, vol.17, no. 2, pp. 139–65.

Clements, S. and Cummings, S. (1991) 'Helplessness and powerlessness: Caring for clients in pain', *Holistic Nursing Practice*, vol. 6, no. 1, pp. 76–85.

Cohen, F. (1980) 'Post surgical pain relief: Patient status and nurses' medication choices', *Pain*, vol. 9, pp. 265–74.

Donovan, M., Dillon, P. and McGuire, L. (1987) 'Incidence and characteristics of pain in a sample of medical–surgical inpatients', *Pain*, vol. 30, pp. 69–78.

Fagerhaugh, S.Y. and Strauss, A. (1977) *Politics of Pain Management*, Menlo Park, CA: Addison-Wesley.

Ferrell, B.A. (1991) 'Pain management in elderly people', *Journal American Pain Society*, vol. 39, pp. 64–73.

Ferrell, B.A., Ferrell, B.R. and Osterwell, D. (1990) 'Pain in the nursing home', *Journal of American Geriatric Society*, vol. 39, pp. 409–14.

Ferrell, B.A., Ferrell, B.R. and Rivera, L. (1995) 'Pain in cognitively impaired nursing home patients', *Journal of Pain and Symptom Management*, vol. 10, pp. 591–5.

Ferrell, B.R., McCaffery, M. and Grant, M. (1991) 'Clinical decision making and pain', *Cancer Nursing*, vol. 14, no. 6, pp. 289–97.

Ferrell, B.R., Whedon, M. and Rollins, B. (1995) 'Pain and quality assessment improvement', *Journal of Nursing Care Quality*, vol. 9, no. 3, pp. 69–85.

Fitzgerald, M. (1994) 'Neurobiology of fetal and neonatal pain', in Wall, P.D. and Melzack, R. (eds) *Textbook of Pain*, 3rd edn, London: Churchill Livingston, pp. 153–63.

Fitzgerald, M. Millard, C. and Macintosh, N. (1989) 'Cutaneous hypersensitivity following peripheral tissue damage in new born infants and its reversal with topical anaesthesia', *Pain*, vol. 39, pp. 31–6.

Francke, A.L., Gassen, B., Abil-Saad, H.H. and Grypdonck, M. (1996) 'Qualitative needs assessment prior to a continuing education program', *The Journal of Continuing Education in Nursing*, vol. 27, no. 1, pp. 39–41.

Frank, L.S. and Miaskowski, C. (1997), 'Measurement of neonatal responses to painful stimuli: A research review', *Journal of Pain and Symptom Management*, vol. 14, pp. 344–78.

Furstenberg, C.T., Ahles, T.A., Whedon, M.B., Pierce, K.L., Dolan, M., Roberts, L. and Silberfarb, P.M. (1998) 'Knowledge and attitudes of health care providers towards lances pain management: A comparison of physicians, nurses, and pharmacist in the state of New Hampshire', *Journal of Pain and Symptom Management*, vol. 15, no. 6, pp. 335–49.

Gaukroger, P. (1992) 'Patient controlled analgesia in children', in Kerr, D. and Thirwell, J. (eds) *Australasian Anaesthesia Book*, Australia & N.Z. College of Anaesthetists, pp. 11–14.

Good, M.J., Brodwin, P.E, Good, B.J. and Kleinman, A. (eds) (1992) *Pain as Human Experience: An Anthropological Perspective*, Berkley: University of California Press.

Graffam, S. (1990) 'Pain content in curriculum—a survey', *Nurse Educators*, vol. 15, no. 1, pp. 20–3.

Greipp, M.E. (1992) 'Under medication for pain: An ethical model', *Advanced Nursing Science*, vol. 15, pp. 44–53.

Gu, X. and Belgrade, M. (1993) 'Pain in hospitalised patients with medical illness', *Journal of Pain and Symptom Management*, vol. 8, no. 17, p. 21.

Illich, I. (1976) *Medical Nemesis: The Exploration of Health*, Hammondsworth: Penguin.

Just, A. (1997) 'The infinite potential of compassion in relieving pain and suffering', *Palliative Care in Australia*, Melbourne: Royal College of Nursing Australia.

Lamacraft, G., Cooper, M.G. and Cavaletta, B.P. (1997) 'Subcutaneous cannulae for morphine boluses in children: Assessment of a technique', *Journal of Pain and Symptom Management*, vol. 13, no. 1, pp. 43–9.

Lander, J. (1990) 'Fallacies and phobias about addiction and pain', *British Journal of Addiction*, vol. 85, no. 6, pp. 803–9.

Langslow, A. (1992) 'Listening but not hearing', *Australian Nurses Journal*, vol. 22, no. 3, pp. 28–30.

Lassell, E.C. (1991) *The Nature of Suffering*, Oxford: Oxford University Press.

Levin, M.L., Berry, J.I. and Leiter, J. (1998) 'Management of pain in terminally ill patients: Physicians reports of knowledge, attitudes and behaviour', *Journal of Pain and Symptom Management*, vol. 15, no. 1, pp. 27–40.

Loeser, J.D. and Cousins, M.J. (1990) 'Contemporary pain management', *The Medical Journal of Australia*, vol. 153, pp. 208–13.

Margolius, F.R., Hudson, K.A. and Michel, Y. (1995) 'Beliefs and perceptions about children in pain: A survey', *Pediatric Nursing*, vol. 21, no. 2, pp. 111–15.

Marks, R.M. and Sachar, E.J. (1973) 'Undertreatment of medical patients with narcotic analgesics', *Annuals Internal Medicine*, vol. 77, pp. 173–81.

McCaffery, M. (1968) *Nursing Practice Theories Related to Cognition, Bodily Pain, and Man-environment Interactions*, Los Angeles: University of California Press.

McCaffery, M. (1979) *Nursing Management of the Patient in Pain*, 2nd edn, Philadelphia: J.B. Lippincott.

McCaffery, M. and Pasero, C. (1999) *Pain: Clinical Manual*, 2nd edn, London, Sydney: Mosby.

McInnes, C. (1976) 'Editorial: Tight-fisted analgesia', *Lancet*, vol. 19, no. 1, p. 1338.

McLeod, G.A., Davies, T.O. and Colvin, J.R. (1995) 'Shaping attitudes to post operative pain relief: The role of the acute pain team', *Journal of Pain and Symptom Management*, vol. 10, no. 1, pp. 30–4.

McQuay, H. and Moore, A. (1998) *Antidepressants in Neuropathic Pain: An Evidence-based Resource for Pain Relief*, Oxford: Oxford University Press.

Meinhart, N. and McCaffery, M. (1983) *Pain: A Nursing Approach in Assessment and Analysis*, Crofts: Appleton Cutway.

Melzack, R. (1983) *Pain Measurement and Assessment*, New York: Raven Press.

Melzack, R. and Wall, P.D. (1965) 'Pain mechanism: A new theory', *Science*, vol. 150, pp. 971–9.

Merskey, H. (1979) 'Pain terms: A list with definitions and notes on usage recommended by the IASP subcommittee on taxonomy', *Pain*, vol. 6, pp. 249–52.

Mersky, H. (ed.) (1986) 'International Association for the Study of Pain. Classification of chronic pain: Description of chronic pain syndromes and definitions of pain terms', *Pain*, Supplement 3, S1–S225.

Miaskowski, C. (1993) 'Current concepts in the assessment and management of acute pain', *Medsurg Nursing*, vol. 2, no. 1, pp. 28–32.

Moynihan, R. (1998) *Too Much Medicine*, Sydney: ABC Books.

National Health and Medical Research Council (NH&MRC) (1989) *Report of the Working Party on Management of Pain*, Canberra: AGPS.

NH&MRC (1999) *Acute Pain Management: Scientific Evidence*, Canberra: Commonwealth of Australia, www.health.gov.au/nhmrc/publicat/pdfcover/cp57covr.htm

Porter, J. and Jick, H. (1980) 'Addiction rare in patients treated with narcotics', *New England Journal of Medicine*, vol. 302, no. 2, p. 123.

Puntillo, K.A. and Weiss, S.J. (1994) 'Pain: Its mediator and associated morbidity in critically ill cardiovascular surgical patients', *Nursing Research*, vol. 43, no. 1, pp. 31–6.

Puntillo, L.A. and Wilkie, D.J. (eds) (1991) *Assessment of Pain in the Critically Ill*, Marylands: Aspen Publications.

Scarry. E. (1985) *The Body in Pain: The Making and Unmaking of the World*, New York: Oxford University Press.

Scott, L.E., Clum, G.A. and Peoples, J.B. (1983) 'Perioperative predictors of post operative pain', *Pain*, vol. 15, pp. 283–93.

Siddall, P.J. and Cousins, M.J. (1997) 'Neurobiology of pain, in Molloy, A.R. and Power, I. (eds) *International Anesthesiology Clinics*, Raven PA: Lippincott.

Siikorski, J. (1994) *Medicine Adrift*, Gold Coast: Pelican Press.

Solute, N. and Cuts, M.D. (1986) 'Analgesia in the acute abdomen', *Annals of the Royal College of Surgeons*, vol. 27, no. 1, pp. 39–41.

Southall, D.P., Cronin, B.C. and Hartmann, H. (1993) 'Invasive procedures in children receiving intensive care', *British Medical Journal*, vol. 306, pp. 560–3.

Taddio, A., Stevens, B. and Craig, K.D. (1997) 'Efficacy and safety of Lidocaine/Prilocaine cream for pain during cicumcision', *New England Journal of Medicine*, vol. 336, pp. 1197–2001.

Tittle, M. and McMillan, S.C. (1994) 'Pain and pain related side effects in an ICV and on a surgical unit: Nurses management', *American Journal of Critical Care*, vol. 3, no. 1, pp. 25–30.

Turner, J.G., Clark, A.J., Gauthier, D.K. and Williams, M. (1998) 'The effect of therapeutic touch on pain and anxiety in burns patients', *Journal of Advanced Nursing*, vol. 28, no. 1, pp. 10–20.

Walding, M.F. (1991) 'Pain, anxiety and powerlessness', *Journal of Advanced Nursing*, vol. 16, pp. 388–97.

Walker, A.C., Tan, L. and George, S. (1995) 'Impact of culture on pain management: An Australian nursing perspective', *Holistic Nursing Practice*, vol. 9, no. 2, pp. 48–57.

Walton, M. (1998) *The Trouble with Medicine*, Sydney: Allen & Unwin.

Warden, S., Carpenter, J.S. and Brockopp, D.Y. (1998) 'Nurses' beliefs about suffering and their management of pain', *International Journal of Palliative Nursing*, vol. 4, no. 1, pp. 21–5.

Weir, R., Roberts, J., Browne, G.B., Crook, J. and Barnes, W. (1990) 'Predictors of narcotic analgesic administration in the first 48 post-operative hours', *Canadian Journal of Nursing Research*, vol. 22, no. 4, pp. 61–73.

Wicks, D. (1999) *Nurses and Doctors at Work*, Sydney: Allen & Unwin.

Zalon, M.L. (1993) 'Nurses assessment of post operative patients pain', *Pain*, vol. 54, pp. 329–34.

Zoltie, N. and Cust, M.D. (1986) 'Analgesia in the acute abdomen', *Annals of Royal College of Surgeons England*, vol. 68, pp. 209–10.

COMMENTARY—CHAPTER 1

Michael Cousins

Isobel Taylor and Shirley Anne Wilson have placed the management of pain in the context that it deserves, namely as a multi-dimensional problem which requires a strong multi-disciplinary approach. In my 30 years of research, clinical work and education in this field, I have seen enormous changes that have provided great potential benefits for patients with severe pain. Thirty years ago very few patients obtained effective relief of pain after surgery, cancer pain relief was really not a priority and it was very early days for the management of chronic non cancer pain, since knowledge was deficient and thus few, if any, patients obtained really effective pain management. There are now major potential improvements representing an extraordinary opportunity: more than 90% of pain after surgery and in association with cancer can be effectively relieved, while more than 75% of patients with chronic non cancer pain can be effectively managed. However, by and large, this is not yet the situation. The authors have defined some of the reasons behind this discrepancy between the possible and the current reality. Although there has been an explosion of knowledge and there is a great need for educational initiatives, it is quite clear that this alone will not allow us to bridge the gap between the possible and reality. The 1988 report of the NH&MRC of Australia on 'The Management of Severe Pain' encapsulated many of the strategies that are needed for a move forward: 'Changes are called for in training, knowledge, attitudes and practices of medical, nursing and allied professionals, along with greater public awareness and expectations in the treatment of pain'.

Taylor and Wilson have made the suggestion that pain needs to be approached as a 'quality issue' and that improvements should be addressed in a manner similar to the implementation of universal precautions against infection. They have hit upon a very key issue here since one of the major failings in pain management has been a lack of a focus on the problem, as exemplified by the frequent absence of any method of documenting patients' pain. Many institutions now use a patient record that tracks visual analogue pain score, sedation score and respiratory rate, as a method of monitoring the patient's pain, efficacy of analgesic measures and side effects resulting from these measures. However, this is but one approach to 'changing attitudes and practices', which will be crucial to realising the advances in pain management that are now possible.

Why should attitudes and practices change? In 1999 the NH&MRC published the evidence based in *Acute Pain Management: Scientific Evidence*. It was noted that the current financial costs of severe unrelieved pain in Australia amount to more than $10 billion annually. The document also provides evidence of adverse outcomes associated with ineffective management of severe pain. Thus there is now very compelling evidence from an economic standpoint that changes in the management of severe pain could produce large financial savings. The Federal Minister for Health in Australia, the Hon. Dr Michael Wooldridge, estimated that at least 25% of costs could be saved by applying best practice. This would result in about $4.8 billion annually of cost savings in Australia. However, with all of this emphasis on financial matters in medicine at the present time, there is a great danger of losing sight of important humanitarian issues which are very effectively brought out by Taylor and Wilson. In my E. A. Rovenstine Memorial Lecture at the Annual Scientific Meeting of the American Society of Anesthesiologists, I described the failure of clinicians to relieve severe pain as being 'torture by omission'. I have also called for pain relief to be recognised by the United Nations as a basic human right. The current list of human rights recognised by the United Nations Declaration includes: freedom from hunger; freedom from thirst; peace without political or other persecution; freedom of speech, press, religion, assembly, mobility; availability of unpolluted food, water and air supply. Few would argue with these as being top priorities, however, it is very difficult to enjoy any of these freedoms if one has unrelenting severe pain.

Thus the relief of severe pain must come close to the top of any list of basic human rights.

Having just returned from the IASP World Congress on Pain which attracted over 6000 registrants, I and others cannot help but be impressed by the explosion of new basic and clinical science knowledge pertinent to this field. And yet, pain is still not emerging as a major societal issue, as it clearly should. The authors of this chapter have quite rightly drawn attention to ethico-legal issues in pain management. It is my contention that any civilised society should put pain management as a very high priority. One would have to have concerns about societies in which relief of pain and suffering, in all age groups, fails to be given appropriate priority. I am very much attracted to the quotation from the ANC's code of ethics that Taylor and Wilson cite. I hope this is taken up by all of those in the health care professions and by society at large. It is interesting to note the judgment in South Australia for negligence in failing to relieve pain. I am aware of another case on the North American continent and I suspect that such cases may play a part in changing societal attitudes, although hopefully this should not be the driving force.

At the end of the romantic era in the 1840s an enormous societal sea-change in attitude occurred towards the relief of pain associated with surgery and child birth. Unfortunately an emphasis on economic matters in health care has, if anything, de-emphasised humanitarian issues in health care. We are now overdue for a return to the type of revolution in societal attitudes that made the acceptance of anaesthesia for surgery and analgesia for child birth such a major contribution to humanity. We are poised to achieve major advances in the relief of acute, chronic and cancer pain, but these potential advances will only be realised with major changes in attitudes and practices.

REFERENCES

NH&MRC (1988) *Management of Severe Pain*, Canberra: AGPS.
NH&MRC (1999) *Acute Pain Management: Scientific Evidence*, Canberra: AGPS.

2 Managing wounds

Keryln Carville

INTRODUCTION

> For us who Nurse, our Nursing is a thing, which, unless we are
> making progress every year, every month, every week, take my word
> for it we are going back (Florence Nightingale 1872).

If ever there was a facet of nursing practice that must reflect the
wisdom expressed here by Miss Nightingale, it is wound management.
As nurses we practice in an exciting age. New information about
wound healing is being generated at an extraordinary rate and
advances in technology have resulted in a plethora of wound management products and devices from which today's practitioners may
choose. Scientific advances have provided wound clinicians with so
many choices that wound management decisions are becoming more
complex and, for some, confusing. In an effort to eliminate confusion
and simplify decision making some nurses limit their wound dressing
choices to a few known favourites and appear reluctant to embrace
the latest technology while others return to traditional practices or
alternatively seek solutions in therapies other than those generally
recognised and accepted in mainstream nursing practice.

The search for the panacea of wound healing has been influenced
by bias, tradition and spiritual beliefs since the earliest of times and
much can be learnt about modern wound management when we review
the practices of the past. We can assume that prehistoric people
recognised that wound healing was aligned with survival and instinc-
tively they would have attempted to stem bleeding and protect the
wound. They would have used substances at hand, such as mud, bark,

leaves and perhaps less desirable substances such as excreta. Paleo-pathological studies on ancient human relics provide evidence of our early ancestors' skill in trepanation, splinting of fractured bones and the use of cautery (Lyons & Petrucelli 1987). Some ancient populations resorted to very creative methods to achieve healing. The Masai tribes in Africa used acacia thorns to approximate wound edges and laced twine between the protruding thorns to promote primary intention. Ancient Indian and South American tribes used termites or beetles for the same purpose, allowing the insects to bite across the edges of a wound. Once anchored in the tissues, the body of the insect was broken off (Haeger 1988). Both practices achieved the same effect as modern day sutures and surgical staples.

Historic documents give insight into past wound healing practices and we learn that they were not all without risk but that some even remain in vogue today. The Pen-tsao (c. 2800 BC), the herbal dossier of the Chinese Emperor Shen Nung, records that wealthy Chinese of that period used elephant skin as a treatment for skin lesions while highly poisonous acontin from the monkshood plant was often recommended for boils and ulcers, with frequent disastrous results. The Edwin Smith Papyrus and Papyri Ebers, Egyptian documents dating back to 1600 BC, suggested cleaning wounds with water which, of course, is still highly recommended today. However, the ancient Egyptians believed the water to have additional therapeutic value if the male member of the household had previously used it for bathing (Haeger 1988).

The Egyptians also used honey, milk and resin adhesives as wound dressings and these have been proven to have a role in modern wound management. The therapeutic value of honey, a traditional favourite for 4000 years, has only been scientifically substantiated in recent times (Harris 1994; Molan 1998). Likewise, milk has been found to contain a variety of cytokines or growth factors that do regulate tissue repair (Cox 1994) and the many adhesive dressings and bandages that we take for granted today trace their descendancy from the Egyptian practice of applying resins to bandages.

The art, or skill, involved in wound care has evolved down through the ages. However, the science of wound healing can be considered a relatively late development. History acknowledges the scientific endeavours of many famous 'ancients' that have influenced our understanding of wounds and healing. Among these are Hippocrates (460–136 BC), known as the 'father of medicine', who listed some astute observations on healing wounds, and Herophilus (335–280 BC), the 'father of Anatomy', who provided an anatomical reference. Celsus

(25 BC–50 AD) bequeathed to us his enduring definition of infection: tumor (swelling), rubor (redness), calor (heat) and dolor (pain) (Haeger 1988; Brown 1992). But it was the scientific discoveries of Hunter, Semmelweis, Pasteur and Lister during the late eighteenth and nineteenth centuries that advanced our understanding dramatically.

John Hunter (1728–93) described healing by primary and secondary intention and expanded on the physiology of wound healing (Brown 1992). Since then, teachers of medicine have educated succeeding generations of doctors in this ever-expanding body of knowledge. Nurses were not so fortunate in receiving such education. To many nurses the science of wound healing remained a mystery for it was rarely taught until the introduction of tertiary institution-based education for nurses. Prior to that, nursing training focused on the rituals of dressing wounds, rather than the science of healing them. Considering nursing is, and has always been, predominantly involved in the care of the patient's integument—either preservation of its integrity or endeavours to promote its repair—this short-coming in earlier nursing education was remiss and supported traditional practices rather than scientific endeavour. However, there is not much evidence to suggest that more informed medical practitioners were also more enlightened when it came to clinical practice.

Enlightenment gradually dawned following George Winter's discovery in 1962 that epithelialisation occurred more speedily in the presence of moisture. Winter's research was published in a one-page report in the journal *Nature*. Although it went largely unnoticed at first, it was without doubt the stimulus for wound research and the development of technology. As a result, today we have an enormous variety of 'new generation' wound care products that promote moist wound healing principles. It could be said that it was during the late 1960s and early 1970s when the art and science of wound management finally merged. Since then there has been more research into wound healing than ever before. Much of this research has challenged the wound care practices of the past and, for some, also the present.

CHALLENGING PRACTICE

During the late 1980s past wound care rituals and traditions were examined in the light of new knowledge and those that could not be substantiated were discarded. Practitioners across all disciplines were gradually exposed to new research and technology that was being rapidly generated. Nurses in particular were at the forefront of change and information was disseminated widely through nursing literature and professional meetings. Often there was confrontation among the traditionalists and revolutionists from both nursing and medical disciplines about the use of moist wound healing, topical antimicrobials (especially the sodium hypochlorites), the use of occlusive dressings, clean instead of sterile equipment and other contentious issues.

Traditionally wounds were kept as dry as possible and were often exposed to sunlight or infra-red lamps in the belief that the presence of moisture would increase the risk of infection in the wound. It was Paracelsus (1493–1541), a Renaissance barber-shop surgeon, who first claimed that wound exudate was nature's balsam and should be left in situ on the wound (Haeger 1988). But his advice went unheeded for centuries until Winter's publication (1962) and the work of Hohn, Pounce and Burton (1977) who were able to demonstrate the antimicrobial effect of wound fluid. A recent resurgence of interest in this 'nature's balsam' has focused on the type and function of the cytokines it contains (Wysocki 1996; Phillips et al. 1998).

Perhaps surprisingly, it has taken people a long time to discover what the animal kingdom had been demonstrating since creation: that the licking of wounds to keep them moist facilitates healing. But people depend on wound dressings to provide a more aesthetic and sociably acceptable option and since the 1970s a plethora of new-generation dressings have come into being bearing a 'moist wound healing' label.

Initially, there was considerable reluctance to embrace this technology, especially those whose practice involved acute surgical wounds. This reluctance was largely due to the fact that the moisture retention dressings were predominately occlusive or semi-occlusive and there was a perception that they would increase the risk of anaerobic infection, particularly in an acute surgical wound. Although this ultimately proved unfounded (Gilchrist & Reed 1989; Hutchinson 1989), it was in the field of chronic wound management that moisture retention dressings were most appreciated first. Not only did these dressings require less frequent changes, they maintained a stable wound temperature. The concept of maintaining a stable wound temperature of around 37°C (Hermans & Bolton 1993; Lock 1979) was a challenge to the wound care ritual of leaving wounds exposed in preparation for medical rounds or dressing teams. The small delays caused to these 'inspection teams' when this practice was discarded in favour of maintaining temperature and promoting mitotic activity in the wound was often interpreted as tardiness on the part of the nurse. Responsibilities and routines were challenged when the scientifically supported move away from antiseptics and frequent wet compress dressings (especially those wet with sodium hypochlorites) favoured the new moisture retention dressings. One nurse manager insisted that the move away from compress dressings would lead to unemployed nurses because they would have nothing to do with their time if they didn't dress wounds!

The conflict over the use of antiseptics on wounds was particularly heated and was stimulated by research during the 1980s that demonstrated the cytotoxic effect of antiseptics on the healing wound (Brennan & Leaper 1985; Lineaweaver et al. 1985). Hospital wards, community settings and the literature became battlefields on which were bandied terms such as negligence and malpractice and lists of detriments to healing from both sides of the antiseptic conflict. Frustrated nurses searched and cited the research literature as well as nursing and common law acts to support the removal of sodium hypochlorite disinfectants from treatment rooms to pan rooms. It took almost a decade before collaboration and consensus on this issue reconciled all practitioners to the fact that, although routine use of antiseptics in healthy wounds is detrimental, there is a therapeutic advantage in the appropriate and prudent use of antiseptics in some infected wounds, particularly those with insufficient vascular status to support systemic infection control.

Aligned with the antiseptic debate was the issue of asepsis in general. Wound cleaning and dressing rituals which were taught and performed with precision though little consensus, were re-examined. Nurses, it appears, could never agree whether wounds should be cleaned from the inside out, or the outside in, from top to bottom or circumferentially. The most creative approach was a zig-zag method of cleaning that adopted most of the previous approaches! It is hard to imagine that, regardless of direction, we really believed that by wiping a few moistened cotton balls over the wound and periwound skin that we could sterilise the wound and protect it from potential contagins, let alone normal skin flora. Gradually we came to realise that the healthy individual lives in harmony with large numbers of resident bacteria. Dry skin flora averages 10 to 1000 bacteria per gram of tissue, with dramatic increases in the bacterial load of moist tissue, saliva or faeces (Lawrence 1992). Resident skin flora will colonise a wound as it does intact skin surfaces, without necessarily being detrimental to healing. A surgical wound is said to be infected if there is a level of bacterial growth of 100 000 (10^5) organisms per gram of tissue with the exception of beta haemolytic Streptococcus, which appears to cause infection at levels lower than 10^5 (Robson 1979; Robson, Stenberg & Heggers 1990). There is evidence, however, that chronic wounds can contain higher levels of bacteria (Gilchrist & Reed 1989; Hutchinson 1989) or greater numbers of different species of bacteria (Trengove et al. 1996) before infection is clinically evident and healing is retarded. It is perhaps a revelation to some to discover that bacteria actually have a positive role to play in healing, for granulation only occurs in the presence of bacteria (Heggers 1998).

Entrenched beliefs and rituals are being challenged. The clean versus sterile wound care debate remains one of the current controversial issues in wound management and yet it is one of the most under-researched. The fact that there is a dearth of research into the use of clean instead of sterile equipment remains a mystery, for the implications to clinical practice and cost-savings are extensive. The meagre amount of research that exists demonstrates no significant difference between a clean or sterile wound dressing technique (Stotts et al. 1997; Wise et al. 1997). However, most practitioners could supply a large amount of anecdotal evidence to support the washing of many wounds and the use of clean instead of sterile dressings. But until there is more credible research to substantiate this practice in all situations, the onus remains on the clinician's ability to assess the person, their wound and their healing environment for compromising factors that warrant the use of sterile equipment.

TOOLS OF THE TRADE

Although the explosion of interest in wound healing and dressing technology was initiated by scientists searching for cellular and biochemical explanations for wound healing, it has been supported and maintained predominantly by the commercial sector in a profit-generated search for the 'perfect dressing'. Gamgee dressings, commonly called combine dressings in Australia, have been surpassed by a continually expanding variety of products and wound pharmaceuticals. In 1993 there were estimated to be over 2000 wound dressings on the market from which the practitioner could choose (Krasner & Rolstad 1993). Today, there are many more that provide an array of options from an ever-expanding variety of generic categories of dressings. Not only are there more brands available within each generic category of dressings but many manufacturers produce more than one dressing within each generic group or use marketing relationships between international companies to expand their product varieties. We now have wound dressings that, in many instances, resemble multi-layered 'club' sandwiches, for they offer many properties or generic characteristics in one product. Some manufacturers even describe their dressings as 'intelligent' and the novice clinician could be forgiven for thinking that one only has to choose that product and the need for ongoing decision making will be eliminated.

In an effort to simplify decision making, some nurses are restricting their choice of dressing products, not taking advantage of the latest technology. Often this restriction is directed by managers who limit available dressing selections in the belief that it will promote cost-containment. Either way it is short-sighted: technology advances, even if practitioners do not. The degree of advancement is evident with the range of topical autologous and exogenous recombinant growth factors, biological dressings and tissue engineering products that are infiltrating the wound care market. The manipulation of human tissue cells to produce cytokines and skin substitutes herald hope for people with chronic wounds or large areas of tissue destruction. As these third generation products become more commercialised and less cost-prohibitive they will make obsolete those dressings we use today.

In the meantime, the informed clinician must be aware that wound management is more than putting on a dressing and that there is no dressing suitable for every wound or every person: the choice of dressing can only be determined after assessing the needs of the person, their wound and their healing environment. All wounds need to be seen as fragile healing environments and healing must not be retarded by wound practices, pharmaceuticals or dressings that traumatise or litter the wound. The onus is on the nurse, therefore, to be skilled in assessment and to understand the 'tools-of-the-trade': the mode of action, contents and contraindications of dressings and devices.

SPECIALISATION

Although the evolution of formalised nursing and medicine are inter-twined and reliant on each other it was to nurses that the task of cleaning and dressing wounds traditionally fell. Florence Nightingale could be considered the first nurse wound specialist for she clearly demonstrated expertise in managing wounded people. Prior to her arrival in Scutari in 1854 there was a death rate among British soldiers of 42% in those hospitalised with wounds and disease, but within the six months following her arrival this was reduced to 2%, mainly as a result of providing better hygiene, nutrition and wound care (Mellish 1984). This was an extraordinary achievement when one considers the dearth of resources Nightingale had at hand.

The tidal wave of professional interest in wound research and technology has seen wound management develop into a highly specialised area of clinical practice with many sub-specialties. Specialisation predominantly involves wound types and practitioners. The diversity and prevalence of wound types are only exceeded by the diversity of both wound treatments and the practitioners who are involved in wound care. Although wound care has always been, and hopefully always will be, a component of nursing care, the role of the clinical nurse specialist or nurse consultant in wound management was an inevitable and natural evolution. This is similar to the development of other clinical nurse specialist roles where knowledge, technology or consumer expectations have expanded well beyond the scope of generalist nursing roles.

It has been claimed that clinical nurse specialists 'know more and more about less and less' (Wade & Moyer 1989). The challenge to this statement is that there is more and more to learn about an ever-expanding field which has outgrown the generalist role. In fact, the specialty of wound management is expanding so rapidly that there are specialists within specialties. The latter relate to the individual clinical practices such as burns and plastics, draining complex wounds, stomal therapy practice and leg ulcer clinics. The specialist role is defined as having several sub-roles of advanced practitioner, educator, consultant, researcher and change agent (Storr 1988). To these must be added the sub-role of clinical manager for there is an expectation that resources used in practice will be managed cost-effectively and distributed equitably. It would be impossible for generalist nurses to fulfil all these responsibilities in addition to their usual burden.

Frequently there is confusion about the defining of specialist and consultant roles. The former is perceived, at least in the British literature, as being an expert practitioner whose role could lead to fragmentation of care as specialisation lays claims to either more nursing care or anatomical functions (Bale 1995; Hollinworth 1993). The consultant role, on the other hand, is perceived to be supportive of the primary practitioner (Hollinworth 1993). Both interpretations are too pedantic and one must question more the way the specialist or consultant—whatever the title—efficiently fulfils all the sub-roles, rather than the title they possess. It is not possible nor is it desirable for a specialist nurse to be responsible for all the wounds within an agency. The major objective of the role is to promote evidence-based practice and collaborative and multi-disciplinary care.

These are also the major objectives of the Australian Wound Management Association which emerged initially as a result of nursing interest, but expanded rapidly to attract medical and allied health professionals. The first national conference specifically on wound management was held in Perth, Western Australia in March 1993 and was aptly titled 'Turning Wound Care Upside Down'. It was at this meeting the need was formally discussed, and a process determined, for establishing a national multi-disciplinary body in wound management. Prior to this, wound management had been seen as a sub-culture of all disciplines and clinical specialties. However, the scientific research presented and the interest generated at this conference demonstrated the need for a unified body to 'spread the word'. Thus, the Australian Wound Management Association became a reality and offered a forum for nursing, medical and allied health professionals to share their interest and expertise in wound management.

The 1990s saw a seemingly unquenchable thirst for education in wound management among nurses at all levels. To satisfy this demand seminars, conferences and courses flourished and nursing literature abounded with related topics. The commercial sector marketed value-added services in the form of educational resources to wound practitioners and some manufacturers even employed their own specialist nurses to provide a credible education service. Surprisingly though, there has been an extremely limited response to addressing this need from most of the nation's schools of nursing; few appear to have recognised the value of dedicated post graduate programs with formalised qualifications in the subject. In many instances clinicians question whether the undergraduate programs are able to keep abreast of the constantly changing clinical scene and adequately prepare new graduates for modern wound management. Is there an expectation that the profession's novices will learn wound management at the bedside, as their forebears did? If so, the presence of a nurse specialist in wound management should be a fundamental requirement in the clinical setting.

COST OF WOUND CARE

The settings in which wounds are cared for are varied and usually relate to the type of wound or acuity of condition and may involve an acute, extended care or community environment. In centuries past, the care of the wounded was largely the responsibility of family, the military or visiting religious orders (Mellish 1984). Early Christian hospitals began as 'houses of hospitality' for the poor (Goldin 1994) and in some instances institutions for isolating the infectious or insane.

The affluent sick or wounded were generally cared for in their own homes.

The mid nineteenth century has been described by some historians as a period of enlightenment that was born of the political, social and scientific revolution that occurred during that century (Mellish 1984). It was a fertile period of development for nursing, medicine and hospitals as establishments of care and learning. The emphasis from home to hospital care became apparent as an economically viable method of maximising health care service and by the mid twentieth century was deeply entrenched as a societal norm for the sick and wounded. The economic rationalism of the 1990s however, resulted in a revival of home health care delivery for all but the most acutely ill. The presence of quite complex wounds presented no barrier to hospital discharge and wound management activity reverted to the community setting in search of less costly alternatives for care (Arnold 1992).

Phrases such as cost-effectiveness and cost-containment were virtually non-existent in Australia's health care settings until the late 1980s (Biscoe 1989), while today these words appear to influence every health care decision, not least of which is wound management. Cost-containment and cost-effectiveness have become buzz-words which complement a vocabulary of new-age terms that have evolved in response to directing care and preventing budget blow-outs. Critical paths, clinical pathways, care-maps, clinical algorithms are but some of these terms used to direct and track quality and cost-effective care. However, regardless of the terminology, these direction and tracking methods traverse many obstacles in mapping anticipated wound healing, for normality is probably the most vital element of any critical path (Tallon 1995); wounds are not normal but are complications of diseases, injury or surgery.

Cost-containment is not necessarily cost-effectiveness. Costs of dressing supplies usually are second to salary costs and frequent dressing changes consume more staff time. Inversely, the move towards disposable dressing materials may have reduced staff time but to their detriment these materials are generally not recyclable or biodegradable, which impacts heavily on environmental costs. Many of the second generation dressings are considerably more expensive when compared to the traditional dry dressings they have replaced. However, dressings with a higher unit cost are generally more cost-effective (Carville & Lewin 1998; Morison 1992) when durability, therapeutic value and comfort are considered. The indirect costs are often not so simple to calculate and should consider the effects of wounds and wounding on such issues as quality of life, maintaining independence and lost work hours (Phillips 1996). The chronicity of the wound reflects not only on the direct costs to the care provider but the indirect costs to the care consumer and the community as a whole. Therefore, it would seem reasonable that dressings that promote faster healing or facilitate return to normal lifestyle should be used regardless of the initial cost.

The true cost of healing wounds is difficult to ascertain but chronic wounds consume more resources and represent the longest episodes of care. Leg ulcers often present as chronic wounds and Baker and Stacey (1994) described a prevalence of 1.1 per 1000 population in an urban Western Australian community. They found that prevalence increased with age, with 91% of those with leg ulcers over 60 years and 58% of the limbs had been ulcerated for more than three months and 24% for a duration of more than two years. Other studies have produced similar findings (Callam et al. 1985; Carville & Lewin 1998; Cornwall, Dore & Lewis 1986).

It is estimated that in the United Kingdom leg ulcer management represents 15 to 50% of community nurse work time and the cost of leg ulcer management to the national budget is £150–600 million per annum (Leaper 1995). In the United States chronic venous leg ulcers are estimated to cost approximately US$40 000 per episode (Capeheart 1996). A survey of patients registered with the Sydney Central Area Health Service demonstrated 200 leg ulcer clients requiring 15% of the nursing time at a cost of $260 000 per week for nursing time alone (Hughes 1997). A survey in Western Australia demonstrated patients with leg ulcers constituted 48% (n=817) of all wounds being managed by the major domicilary nursing service and mean healing times and costs of healing were considerably higher than other wound types surveyed (Carville & Lewin 1999).

Cost should not be the only parameter used to evaluate practice. A systematic clinical audit of actual practices is suggested as a means of monitoring and evaluating quality outcomes (Burnett & Winyard 1998; Morison 1992). One such clinical audit to determine the number and type of all wounds being managed in the community in Western Australia provided information regarding the management of 1699 wounds and resulted in the development of a comprehensive standard of assessment for the person with a wound and education and clinical competency programs for nurses (Carville & Lewin 1998). If we are to optimise patient outcomes and contain health care costs we must be able to evaluate our standards of practice and ensure that they are evidence-based and efficiently use the resources available.

CONCLUSION

Wound care—the simple art of dressing a wound—has evolved into wound management—the art and science of assessment and management of the person, their wound and their healing environment. This evolution has not occurred without confrontation and casualties. It appears that, with few exceptions, more has been done through the ages to retard wound healing, albeit unintentionally, than promote it. Unlike many of our ancestors, our wound management practices can no longer reflect ignorance for we live in an era where we are continually confronted by information from the professional and secular media. This exposure firmly places the onus on all practitioners to examine their ways of operating and to discard those practices that can't be substantiated scientifically. More importantly, our nation's finite health dollar and increasing health consumer expectations demand compliance.

There is great promise for advancement in wound healing technology. There will be a greater focus on tissue engineering and the use of cytokine impregnated products and biological dressings which will eventually make most of the dressings we presently use obsolete. More importantly, there will be scientific advances in medical diagnostics, treatment and genetic manipulation that will eradicate many of the metabolic, vascular and auto-immune disorders that currently predispose to many wounds and delays in healing. We have much to look forward to as practitioners in wound management. But may we always be mindful of the fact that just as we challenge yesterday's practices today, future practitioners will no doubt challenge today's practices tomorrow.

REFERENCES

Arnold, N. (1992) 'A study of wound healing in home care', *Ostomy/Wound Management*, vol. 38, no. 7, pp. 38–44.

Baker, S., and Stacey, M. (1994) 'Epidemiology of chronic leg ulcers in Australia', *Australian and New Zealand Journal of Surgery*, vol. 64, pp. 258–61.

Bale, S. (1995) 'The role of the clinical nurse specialist within the health-care team', *Journal of Wound Care*, vol. 4, no. 2, pp. 86–7.

Biscoe, G. (1989) 'The future: Planning reformation, uncertainty', in Gray, G. and Pratt, R. (eds) *Issues in Australian Nursing 2*, Melbourne: Churchill Livingstone, pp. 83–97.

Brennan, S. and Leaper, D. (1985) 'The effect of antiseptics on healing: A study using the rabbit ear chamber', *British Journal of Surgery*, vol. 72, no. 10, pp. 780–2.

Brown, H. (1992) 'Wound healing research through the ages', in Cohen, K., Diegelmann, R.

and Lindblad, W. (eds) *Wound Healing Biochemical & Clinical Aspects*, Philadelphia: W.B. Saunders Company, pp. 5–18.

Burnett, A. and Winyard, G. (1998) 'Clinical audit at the heart of clinical effectiveness', *Journal of Quality Clinical Practice*, vol. 18, no. 1, pp. 3–19.

Callam, M., Ruckley, C., Harper, D. and Dale, J. (1985) 'Chronic ulceration of the leg: Extent of the problem and provision of care', *British Medical Journal*, vol. 290, pp. 1855–56.

Capeheart, J. (1996) 'Chronic venous insufficiency: A focus on prevention of venous ulceration', *Journal of Wound, Ostomy and Continence Nursing*, vol. 23, no. 4, pp. 227–34.

Carville, K. and Lewin, G. (1998) 'Caring in the community: A wound prevalence survey', *Primary Intention*, vol. 6, no. 2, pp. 54–62.

Carville, K. and Lewin, G. (1999) 'Costs of wound care in the community', unpublished report, Perth: Silver Chain Nursing Association.

Cornwall, J., Dore, C. and Lewis, J. (1986) 'Leg ulcers: Epidemiology and aetiology', *British Journal of Surgery*, vol. 73, no. 9, pp. 693–6.

Cox, D. (1994) 'Milk growth factors', *Journal of Wound Care*, vol. 3, no. 1, pp. 47–8.

Gilchrist, B. and Reed, C. (1989) 'The bacteriology of chronic venous ulcers treated with occlusive hydrocolloid dressings', *British Journal of Dermatology*, vol. 121, pp. 337–44.

Goldin, G. (1994) *Work of Mercy: A Picture History of Hospitals*, Ontario: Boston Mills Press.

Haeger, K. (1988) *The Illustrated History of Surgery*, London: Harold Starke.

Harries, R. and Robson, M. (1997) 'The chronic wound: Definitions and clinical trials', *Primary Intention*, vol. 5, no. 4, pp. 8–13.

Harris, S. (1994) 'Honey for the treatment of superficial wounds: A case report and review', *Primary Intention*, vol. 5, no. 4, pp. 8–13.

Heggers, J. (1998) 'Defining infection in chronic wounds: Does it matter?', *Journal of Wound Care*, vol. 7, no. 8, pp. 389–92.

Hermans, M. and Bolton, L. (1993) 'Air exposure versus occlusion: Merits and disadvantages of different dressings', *Journal of Wound Care*, vol. 2, no. 6, pp. 362–5.

Hohn, D., Pounce, B. and Burton, R. (1977) 'Antimicrobial systems of the surgical wound', *American Journal of Surgery*, vol. 133, no. 5, pp. 597–600.

Hollinworth, H. (1993) 'The specialist nurse in wound management', *Journal of Wound Care*, vol. 2, no. 2, 114–16.

Hughes, J. (1997) 'Ulcer treatment "largely ineffective"', *Medical Observer*, 16 May, p. 5.

Hutchinson, J. (1989) 'Prevalence of wound infection under occlusive dressings: A collective survey of reported research', *Wounds: A Compendium of Clinical Research and Practice*, vol. 1, no. 2, pp. 123–32.

Krasner, D. and Rolstad, B. (1993) 'The ABC of wound care dressings', *Ostomy/Wound Management*, vol. 39, no. 8, pp. 66–86.

Lawrence, W. (1992) 'Clinical management of nonhealing wounds', in Cohen, K., Diegelmann, R. and Lindblad, W. (eds) *Wound Healing Biochemical & Clinical Aspects*, Philadelphia: W.B. Saunders Company, pp. 541–61.

Lazarus, G., Cooper, D., Knighton, D., Margolis, D., Pecoraro, R., Rodeheaver, G. and Robson, M. (1994) 'Definitions and guidelines for assessment of wounds and evaluation of healing', *Archives of Dermatology*, vol. 130, pp. 489–93.

Leaper, D. (1995) 'The management of venous ulcers—the medical and surgical options', *Journal of Wound Care*, vol. 4, no. 10, pp. 477–80.

Lineaweaver, M., Howard, R., Soucy, D., McMorris, S., Freeman, C., Crain, C., Robertson, J. and Rumley, T. (1985) 'Topical antimicrobial toxicity', *Archives of Surgery*, vol. 120, no. 3, pp. 267–70.

Lock, P. (1979) *The Effects of Temperature on Mitotic Activity at the Edge of Experimental Wounds*, Kent, UK: Lock Laboratories Research.

Lyons, A. and Petrucelli, R. (1987) *Medicine: An Illustrated History*, New York: Abradale Press, Harry N. Abrams, Inc.

Mellish, J. (1984) *A Basic History of Nursing*, Durban: Butterworth Publishers.

Molan, P. (1998) 'A brief review of honey as a clinical dressing', *Primary Intention*, vol. 6, no. 4, pp. 148–58.

Morison, M. (1992) 'Quality assurance and wound care in the community', *Ostomy/Wound Management*, vol. 38, no. 8, pp. 38–44.

Nightingale, F. (1872) 'Addresses to the Probationer Nurses in the Nightingale Fund School at St Thomas's Hospital 1872–1900' in Baly, M. (1997) *As Miss Nightingale Said . . .*, 2nd edn, London: Bailliere Tindall.

Phillips, T. (1996) 'Cost-effectiveness in wound care', *Ostomy/Wound Management*, vol. 42, no. 1, pp. 56–9.

Phillips, T., Al-Amoudi, H., Leverkus, M. and Park, H. (1998) 'Effect of chronic wound fluid on fibroblasts', *Journal of Wound Care*, vol. 7, no. 10, pp. 527–32.

Robson, M. (1979) 'Infection in the surgical patient: An imbalance in the normal equilibrium', *Clinics in Plastic Surgery*, vol. 6, no. 4, pp. 493–503.

Robson, M., Stenberg, B. and Heggers, J. (1990) 'Wound healing alterations caused by infection', *Clinics in Plastic Surgery*, vol. 17, no. 3, pp. 485–92.

Storr, G. (1988) 'The clinical nurse specialist: From the outside looking in', *Journal of Advanced Nursing*, vol. 13, no. 2, pp. 265–72.

Stotts, N., Barbour, S., Griggs, K., Bouvier, B., Buhlman, L., Wipke-Tevis, D. and Williams, D. (1997) 'Sterile verses clean technique in postoperative wound care of patients with open surgical wounds: A pilot study', *Journal of Wound, Ostomy and Continence Nursing*, vol. 24, no. 1, pp. 10–18.

Tallon, R. (1995) 'Critical paths for wound care', *Advances in Wound Care*, vol. 8, no. 1, pp. 26–33.

Trengove, N., Stacey, M., McGechie, D., Stingemore, N. and Mata, S. (1996) 'Qualitative bacteriology and leg ulcer healing', *Journal of Wound Care*, vol. 5, no. 6, pp. 277–80.

Wade, B. and Moyer, A. (1989) 'An evaluation of clinical nurse specialists: Implications for education and the organisation of care', *Senior Nurse*, vol. 9, no. 9, pp. 11–16.

Winter, G. (1962) 'Formation of the scab and the rate of epithelialisation of superficial wounds in the skin of the young domestic pig', *Nature*, vol. 193, pp. 293–4.

Wise, L., Hoffman, J., Grant, L. and Bostrom, J. (1997) 'Nursing wound care survey: Sterile and nonsterile glove choice', *Journal of Wound, Ostomy & Continence Nursing*, vol. 24, no. 3, pp. 144–50.

Wyscoki, A. (1996) 'Wound fluids and the pathogenesis of chronic wounds', *Journal of Wound, Ostomy & Continence Nursing*, vol. 23, no. 6, 283–90.

COMMENTARY—CHAPTER 2

Tal Ellis

Wound management has changed enormously over the last 30 years. The ground breaking work by George Winter and others since the early 1960s has resulted in a new understanding of healing and healing enhancement methods. More recently the explosion in wound pharmaceuticals has provided practitioners with a vast choice of treatment options and methods, giving rise to much debate and conjecture over which options are best under differing circumstances. In the context of this changing healthscape Keryln Carville's chapter is important and relevant. Important because it raises and discusses issues that are meaningful, issues that practitioners frequently face. Relevant because the opinions expressed are representative of a significant body of opinion among those who work and research within the field of wound management.

It is apparent that there has been, and still is, some degree of folklore surrounding the teaching and performance of wound management. Traditions, individual interpretations, institutional bias and political factors, in addition to science and researched clinical practice, have all contributed to a plethora of ideas concerning wound management. As a consequence, the notion of evidence based practice in wound management has been relatively slow to evolve. Throughout health and medical practice this ideology is becoming pre-eminent and it represents a significant challenge to those involved in the care of people with wounds to adapt practice accordingly. While this challenge will fall largely in the domain of the specialist practitioner, generalists who practice in the field will need to embrace the ideology in order to ensure that their practice is appropriate and valuable to their clients.

The issues raised by Carville are indeed those that currently confront nurses and represent significant practice and educational challenges for us now and in the future. Through well designed research, practitioners and academics need to advance wound management knowledge and practice at the clinical level so that, through ownership of the change process, better care outcomes can be achieved.

3 Nurse Practitioners

Amanda Adrian & Jane O'Connell

INTRODUCTION

Nurse practitioners are increasingly being identified as legitimate providers of health services throughout the world (American Nurses Association 1993b; Brown & Grimes 1993; Haines 1993; Iliffe 1994; NSW Department of Health 1993; NSW Department of Health 1995; Safriet 1992; Waller 1998). The emergence of the role of 'nurse practitioners' has tended to occur where a clear need arises. This may be because there are no other providers of timely health services or because health consumers are seeking alternatives to their customary health service providers. Many reasons can be attributed to the lack of adequate or appropriate health care, including geographic, economic, social or cultural isolation.

The semantic debate or the 'naming'

The term 'nurse practitioner' remains controversial. For example, a Canadian discussion paper on nurse practitioners (Haines 1993) shows that the issue of definition has provoked comments that are remarkably similar to those noted in Australia. Two of these are that:

- all nurses are practitioners of nursing
- 'practitioner' is a term that has been historically reserved for doctors.

The *Lamp* editorial of August 1994 emerged in response to an interesting aspect of the Nurse Practitioner Project conducted in New

South Wales. The Project has led to a debate within the profession of nursing about 'advanced practice' for nurses. On the one hand there are nurses who argue that the Project was not adventurous enough; while on the other hand there are those who thought otherwise.

This debate is healthy as it challenges the nursing profession to focus on key issues, develop the capacity to research and articulate the evolution going on within the profession. As more creative ways are developed to deliver consumer-focused quality health services, the traditional picture of the nurse, the doctor and the patient is being transformed. The shift from an essentially 'provider driven' system of health service delivery to a more 'consumer driven' system, with recognition of an individual's rights to be informed and make personal choices, has meant that previously entrenched attitudes are having to be seriously examined. These include the traditional ethical, cultural and structural dogma and doctrine of the professions in health. For example, Bartholome describes the 'parentalism' (Bartholome 1993, pp. 19–20), a hybrid of the 'paternalism' of medicine, and the 'maternalism' of nursing, that has directed the nature of the relationships that health professionals have built with their patients in the past.

All these influences are reflected in the radical changes in the organisation and culture of the nursing profession—changes that include: the way nurses are educated; the development of a Code of Ethics and a Code of Conduct; the evolution of nursing research; the development of competencies for nurses; the influence of feminism and equal opportunity policy and legislation; and the recognition of the need to define what it is we do as nurses, rather than what it is we do not do as nurses. These are all having an undeniable effect on the shape of what we 'know' as nursing.

There are great pitfalls with the way nurses are currently labelling the evolutionary stages through which the profession is progressing. For example, the terms 'extended role' and 'advanced practice' should give rise to uneasiness. When nurses talk of 'extended roles', of 'advanced practice' and 'nurse practitioners', they are not talking about being 'new age' doctors or 'new age' anything else (Buhagier 1992; Nelson 1992). Nurses must be clear that they are talking about the practice of nursing. Perhaps nurses have done themselves a disservice by using adjectives such as 'extended', 'advanced' and 'independent' when talking of nursing practice—the implication being that nurses are moving out of clearly designated nursing territory. One of the hazards of not defining clearly what it is that nurses do, and the lingering, detrimental impact of the period of negative definition where 'non-nursing duties' were espoused, is that, by default, nurses seem to have had to go into a reclamation phase. This can easily be interpreted as poaching on other professionals' ground.

The international scene

Ford and Silver in Colorado advanced the nurse practitioner movement in the United States with the inception of the 'Colorado Paediatric Nurse Practitioner and Associate Program' in 1965. Dr Henry Silver and Professor of Nursing, Loretta Ford, in an example of true medical/ nursing collaboration, saw a need for a program to train nurse practitioners. The model was created to expand the scope of nursing without altering its essential nature. At that time, four trends in society and nursing were emerging in the United States concurrently (Ford 1982):

- new conceptualisations about the nature of nursing and health were beginning to appear
- graduate education in nursing was redirecting its focus to clinical specialty majors
- the focus of nursing research was shifting from studies of educational processes and programs and of the nurse as a person and professional, to investigations into clinical practice problems and inquiry into the delivery of health services, and
- hospital costs were soaring with increased instances of cost control mechanisms being implemented.

Professor Betty Anderson from the University of Western Sydney, while delivering her paper on 'The Practitioner Role' for the NSW College of Nursing Annual Oration in 1990, talked of a 'climate ripe for innovation'. She challenged those present to carry out a mental inventory and consider if the nursing profession and the health system in New South Wales had arrived at the juncture described above, ready to develop a successful role for nurse practitioners.

There is extensive international literature focusing on the role and function, the acceptability, cost effectiveness and safety of nurse practitioners. In December 1986, a report from the US Congressional Office of Technology Assessment on nurse practitioners was published. The overall content of the report was very favourable, finding that the care provided by nurse practitioners was of a high standard. Nurses exhibited more personal interest, provided more information, more services such as health promotion, client education and psychosocial support and had better communication, counselling and interviewing skills than other health care providers.

The nurse practitioner role is well established in Canada, with a recognised role being described as far back as 1972. A randomised trial (the Burlington Trial) of the utilisation of nurse practitioners conducted within Ontario in 1972 concluded that: '. . . a nurse practitioner can provide first-contact primary clinical care as safely and effectively, with as much satisfaction to patients as a family physician' (Spitzer et al. 1974, p. 255). The history and evolution of nurse practitioners in Canada was, until the mid 1990s, very much dictated by the waxing and waning of physician supply. In times of surplus, nurse practitioners often found themselves professionally isolated, usually in remote geographical and practice areas (Haines 1993, p. 17; Morewood-Northrop 1994; Van Der Horst 1992). Since 1994 all ten of the university nursing schools in the province of Ontario have offered a nurse practitioner program. Ontario officially recognised the role of nurse practitioners, with the third reading of Bill 127, in June 1997 (Ontario Legislative Assembly, Toronto, Canada). This legislation is intended to allow nurse practitioners to work to their fullest capacity and enable consumers to have wider access to high quality cost-effective health care providers (Registered Nurses' Association of Ontario 1997).

In many countries the role of nurses and nurse practitioners in providing primary or basic health care is very much a necessity and ever developing. Belize, a country in Central America with a population of 217 000, responded to a serious shortage of psychiatrists with the development of a new role, the Psychiatric Nurse Practitioner (PNP). A training program offered by Memorial University School of Nursing in St John's, Newfoundland was conducted over ten months. The evaluation of the role confirmed that: the PNPs were competent to provide community psychiatric care; families and patients were satisfied with the care received; and that the role had developed appropriately (Land 1998).

Rural nurses in Chile carry out public health programs and supervise the work of auxiliary nurses. While these nurses are not described as nurse practitioners, they are highly significant to the delivery of community health services, and without them, basic health care for the community would not be possible (Land 1998).

Some Caribbean countries have had family nurse practitioners for at least 15 years but are yet to pass specific legislation to support the role of nurse practitioners (Land 1998).

The New Zealand Department of Health commissioned a report on nurse practitioners in 1986. The report concluded that with the increasing emphasis on primary health care, nurses can make a significant contribution (Brash 1986). Since that time there is evidence that nurse practitioner services in New Zealand have been evolving across practice settings with the support of initiatives led by the New Zealand Nursing Council and the Nurse Executives of New Zealand (Jacobs 1998).

The opportunity to develop individualised advanced practice programs/roles within specialties has led to a significant degree of variation across the United Kingdom. While professional bodies are trying to formalise many programs and roles, the fact that they have developed in an ad hoc way, driven by one-off need, has made regulation, accreditation and standards difficult to control. Key policy initiatives in health care in the United Kingdom, including responsiveness to the Patient's Charter (Department of Health 1995), changes in service arrangements, reduction in junior doctors' hours and enhancements to primary care services, contributed to the blossoming and variety of 'advanced' practice roles (Waller 1998). Many roles were designed to fill service gaps and as substitutions for other service providers, and were moulded to fit the required purpose. The title, role and function of nurse practitioners have no formal policy or regulatory framework, affording many nurses the opportunity to call themselves 'nurse practitioners'. For consumers and the health system this can lead to confusion and misunderstanding. The National Health Service reforms in the United Kingdom of the late 1990s may provide an opportunity to look at nurse practitioner roles across the whole health system by reviewing role developments that have resulted from key policy initiatives in health care delivery at a national level (Waller 1998).

THE AUSTRALIAN EXPERIENCE

Many nurses in Australia had begun to describe themselves as nurse practitioners by the early 1990s. However, not much had changed in the environment in which they practiced. There remain few opportunities for remuneration other than by direct billing of clients. Until the passing of the *Nurses Amendment (Nurse Practitioners) Act 1998* (NSW) nurses have had no direct rights to prescribe medications. Myth and policy prohibitions surround the ordering of investigations such as x-rays and pathology tests where legislation does not preclude this practice. The controversial topic of liability and indemnity has not been comprehensively tackled. Nor, until the passing of the historic *Nurses Amendment (Nurse Practitioners) Act* in New South

Wales, had the term nurse practitioner entered the formal structures of nurse education, accreditation, certification or registration.

Until recently there had been a paucity of research or literature relating to the role in Australia. However, there was strong anecdotal evidence that nurses, through necessity and choice, had been providing comprehensive and expert primary care, midwifery services, mental health services, women's health services and public health services (to name only a few) to the Australian community for many years. The Nurse Practitioner Project conducted in New South Wales between 1990 and 1998 was a significant marker in the research and development of the nurse practitioner role in Australia.

States and territories in Australia have been watching the NSW Nurse Practitioner Project carefully and most have now begun a local implementation project. A number are directly based on the findings of the New South Wales research. Given the federal system and the state-based organisation of many health services and regulation of health professionals, if the lessons from New South Wales are to be heeded, the most difficult aspect of implementing the different models of nurse practitioner services will be in negotiating with the local key stakeholders.

Politics and posturing: Floodgates, slopes and wedges

Australian experiences reinforce the evidence that difficulties arise when any public discussion begins about legitimising the role and providing nurse practitioners with the necessary legislative and policy framework in which the autonomy of their decision making can be recognised and approved (Napier 1996; NSW Department of Health 1993; NSW Department of Health 1995). The barriers in Australia have included the medical profession's continuing fierce belief in their primal and central role in the provision of health services. This often prevents the most rational of them seeing that an alternative service provider may be able to offer a safe, cost effective service that meets consumers' needs. Underlying this is the ever present and only ever whispered matter of 'turf'. This is a prevailing and difficult subject that requires an enormous amount of energy and political savvy when dealing with it. Any attempt to challenge the ambit that the medical profession views as its own is seen as poaching and is met with a ferocious, very effective, yet fundamental political response.

The Nurse Practitioner Project conducted in New South Wales epitomised the tensions that exist between the ideal of 'collaboration' in the provision of health services and the rather sordid reality of 'competition' from the commencement of Stage 1 in 1990. Extraordinary examples of collaboration were matched by hysterical and defensive reactions to a perception that the Project constituted an invasion of professional (and commercial) territory. Often shrouded in the mystical verbiage of 'safety', 'public interest', 'ethics', 'professionalism', 'competence' and other such emotive terms, the political and the commercial were very much in evidence throughout the three stages of the Project up to the 'roll-out' now occurring. Nurses continue to be surprised by the critical and acrimonious response of the medical profession, from whom they would have expected much more collegial understanding and support in their attempts to better meet the health needs of the greater community. It is a difficult political lesson to learn.

Underlying the stages of the Nurse Practitioner Project, and continuing to be promulgated by some critics, have been assertions that have been difficult to rebut. These are identifiable as the theories of the 'floodgates' and 'the thin edge of the wedge'. Like the 'slippery slope' argument these are insidious and damaging despite the strong evidence supporting the safety and veracity of the nurse practitioner role, in that they have such a strong superficial logic. The 'floodgates' version involves the rather misguided view that, once legitimised, nurse practitioners will proliferate and take over the world! This ignores the fundamental truth that not all registered nurses wish to be nurse practitioners. The evidence from the United States confirms that only a small proportion of registered nurses choose to undertake the additional educational and experiential development required of a nurse practitioner (McGrath in NSW Department of Health 1993).

Each of the recommendations in the *Nurse Practitioner Project Stage 3: Final Report of the Steering Committee* flowed out of issues, hot debate and hard won resolution, based upon the findings of the research and, unavoidably, the values and ethics of the parties around the table and political lobbying. While the Nurse Practitioner Project was a significant landmark in nursing professional history, it was also a significant marker in the political 'blooding' of the profession.

Independence or autonomy?

It is interesting that it was very early in the Nurse Practitioner Project that the issue of 'independence' was raised in relation to nurse practitioners; that is, *before* the debate was broadened to include the medical profession, consumers, policy and legal advisers. In common parlance even today, the term 'independent nurse practitioners' has continued to be used inappropriately in relation to the New South Wales initiatives. Consensus was reached before the release of any public documents that the adjective 'independent' should be dropped when referring to nurse practitioners. Why? Clearly, it was provocative, hampering the debate and was one of the points that was attracting the most virulent response. But, probably more importantly, it was agreed that the provision of health care is by nature, interdependent. It is clearly recognised that collaboration between health professionals is fundamental to the provision of quality health services, whether in outback Australia where the collaboration and consultation may take place via telephone, radio, facsimile or the internet, or in a high level intensive care unit in a tertiary referral centre.

The issue of 'autonomy', that is, the ability and capacity to make decisions (including a decision to seek advice or to refer on), to act on those decisions and be accountable for those decisions was seen as subtly different from the notion of 'independent'. The clinical decision making capacity of the nurses working in a nurse practitioner role was one of the primary research questions of the pilot projects that made up Stage 3 of this Project.

Education of nurse practitioners

Education of nurse practitioners is another area that the NSW Nurse Practitioner Project Stage 3 Steering Committee grappled with at length. While the Committee was not prescriptive about the recommendations in this area, a huge challenge has been issued to education providers and health services. The challenge is to develop and enable attendance at programs that are accessible, relevant and sufficiently rigorous to ensure that registered nurses wishing to work in services that clearly demand the skills, knowledge, attitudes and experience attributable to this level of expert nursing practice, have the opportunity to develop these attributes. The immensity of this demand becomes evident when one looks, for example, at the need for the greater proportion of remote area nurses to have high level nursing practice competencies. These are necessary in order to provide the broad range of primary health care services in places where communications are, at best, unreliable, and often in places where medical practitioners do not go.

The richness of the populations and the variety of clinical assessment and management skills and knowledge that nurse practitioners need are also fertile grounds for creativity in the education models that are developed. The defining of clinical areas of midwifery through primary care to nursing in the palliative care, sexual health, mental health and drug and alcohol arenas is but one of the dimensions. Consumer dimensions such as domestic status (e.g. homelessness), gender, Aboriginality, ethnicity and language, rural or urban environments add to the complexity of the educational experiences that will be required by nurse practitioners. For the Stage 3 Steering Committee to have prescribed that a specific tertiary certificate, diploma or degree is required for a registered nurse to be accredited as a nurse practitioner would have ignored the need for the nursing profession and the educational sector to explore, debate and investigate the best options across the professional spectrum where nurse practitioners may provide quality health services.

SCOPE FOR NURSE PRACTITIONER CLINICAL PRACTICE IN AUSTRALIA

'The NP [nurse practitioner] was very professional but also caring with obvious years of knowledge and practice' (NSW Nurse Practitioner Project 1995). 'I felt as though it was unnecessary to take up the doctor's time on a relatively minor complaint' (NSW Pilot Project Report 1995). There were many positive patient responses to the availability of nurse practitioners highlighted in the pilot project research of Stage 3 of the Nurse Practitioner Project. The ongoing debate on the future for nurse practitioners has mainly focused on the discourse between the nursing and medical bodies. However the consumer response and discussion is extremely important. The public support of nurses is confirmed annually as opinion polls in New South Wales show that the public have the highest degree of confidence and trust in nurses as a professional group (*Bulletin* Morgan Poll 1999). Nurses repeatedly score higher than lawyers and doctors, so it was no surprise that the nurse practitioner role was well received by the public. Patient satisfaction surveys conducted in conjunction with many of the pilot projects in New South Wales also support this assertion. Additionally, these surveys reveal that people appreciated the reduction in waiting time for care at many of the pilot sites.

'Excellent use of resources and available staff' (NSW Nurse Practitioner Project 1995). Many people followed up their positive remarks by recommending that more nurse practitioners should be used to expand the service. The high degree of consumer satisfaction with the services provided by nurse practitioners was indicative of the overall outcomes of the study.

Despite this, another ambiguous issue arose in the research that is important. It is the lack of community understanding of what nursing is. Most would believe they have a good understanding of nursing, but like many nurses, they are unable to articulate their understanding of the scope of the role of nursing. The research into this very question is in its infancy and the discourse and narrative traditions to describe the role are only just being identified. Virginia Henderson spent most of her professional career attempting to describe nursing in an environment of constant social change. She recognised the difficulties inherent in describing a role performed globally, but shaped so strongly by the many add-on layers of the cultural, economic and political influences of each nation, region and local area (Henderson 1978).

For nurses working in the role of nurse practitioners in the pilot research sites in New South Wales, the experience was positive and rewarding. The role identity was strong, due to firm understanding by that group of expert nurses and because the pilot framework was clearly defined. There were many interesting observations made by the nurse practitioners, including 'patient ownership', professional boundaries and professional accountability and responsibility. Professional boundaries have always overlapped in health care and have tended to have intuitive edges with the health professionals developing a workable understanding of them. The legitimisation of the nurse practitioner role has seen these boundaries further blur, resulting in anxiety and confusion for many health professionals (Doyal 1998; Waller 1998).

The continuum of change, expressed in the development of the nurse practitioner role, is not new. The preparation and function of a registered nurse broadened and evolved dramatically in each decade of the twentieth century. There is no reason to assume that this evolution will not continue as the health needs of the community change during the twenty-first century. Nurse practitioners are a manifestation of this progress.

Nurses involved in the research in New South Wales identified that the personal experience of being able to work fully to ones' capabilities was remarkable, after many years of feeling constrained and invisible. It was satisfying to be recognised and 'allowed' to work somewhat autonomously, without having to continuously defer to a doctor for permission to perform a role that for many is very comfortable. This comfort arises from the individual's depth of knowledge and experience, enabling them to make competent, informed clinical decisions, confident in the outcomes for the people to whom they are providing care (Concord Repatriation General Hospital/Royal Prince Alfred Hospital 1994).

One of the concerns of resident medical officers (RMOs) at one pilot site during the Nurse Practitioner Project was that their workload would increase because they had to 'supervise' the nurse practitioner. In fact, even in this research phase where a review of the clinical decisions of nurse practitioners was required as part of the research methodology, there was evidence that the workload of the RMO was reduced. Surveys conducted at that time showed that 25% of medical respondees perceived a decrease in workload as an outcome of the nurse practitioner pilot project at that site (NSW Nurse Practitioner Project 1995).

CONCLUSION

While much early research on nurse practitioner services appears to concentrate on primary care, it has become increasingly common, particularly in the United States, for nurse practitioners to practice in tertiary care facilities in acute care settings:

> the nurse practitioner model of practice was originally designed to meet the needs of ambulatory populations to maintain health, yet there remain tremendous unmet needs in acute and long-term care settings for which nurses have the potential, opportunity and accountability to respond (Ford 1979).

The advent of trauma nurse practitioners and neonatal intensive care nurse practitioners in the United States should indicate that the development from purely primary care settings to tertiary settings is a natural evolution. Already there is some activity and interest in the tertiary sector in Australia. For example, John Hunter Hospital in Newcastle (NSW) undertook a feasibility pilot study in the neonatal intensive care unit in the mid 1990s. However, caution is needed to ensure that the nurse practitioner role is developed because of its intrinsic value in providing quality, feasible, safe, effective and afford-able health services, and not developed only as a response to gap filling, cheap doctor substitution or professional self interest.

Strengthening health systems through nursing can lead to an increased coverage of basic health services for those most in need. Nurses are already established in the health workforce in significant numbers and are often working to provide care to diverse populations.

The law in Australia is relatively straightforward—nurses are responsible for their actions on a daily basis, to extend their scope of practice will not diminish their accountability.

REFERENCES

American Nurses' Association (1993a) 'Advanced practice nursing: A new age in health care', *Nursing Facts*, PR–1135M 8/93, Washington DC.

American Nurses' Association (1993b) *Scope of Practice for Nurse Practitioners*, Washington DC.

American Nurses' Association (1993c) *Advanced Practice Nursing: State Legislative Survey*, Washington DC.

Bartholome, W.G. (1993) 'A revolution in understanding: How ethics has transformed health care decision making', *Bioethics News*, January, vol. 12, no. 2.

Brash, J. (1986) *The Independent Nurse Practitioner in New Zealand*, Department of Health Nursing section, Workforce Development, December.

Brown, S.A. and Grimes, D.E. (1993) 'Executive summary', *A Meta-Analysis of Care, Clinical Outcomes and Cost Effectiveness of Nurses in Primary Care Roles: Nurse Practitioners and Midwives*, American Nurses' Association, Washington DC.

Buhagiar, T. (1992) 'General practice must repel the invaders', *Australian Doctor*, September, vol. 11.

Bulletin, The Morgan Poll (1999) 'The professions we trust the most', 29 June, p. 35.

Concord Repatriation General Hospital/Royal Prince Alfred Hospital (1994) *Final Report on the Emergency Department Nurse Practitioner Pilot Project*, NSW Department of Health.

Department of Health (UK) (1995) *The Patient's Charter*, rev. edn, London: Department of Health.

Doyal, L. (1998) 'Crossing professional boundaries', *Nursing Management*, vol. 5, no. 4, pp. 8–10.

Ford, L. (1979) 'A nurse for all settings: The nurse practitioner', *Nursing Outlook*, vol. 27, no. 8, pp. 516–21.

Ford, L. (1982) 'Nurse practitioners: History of a new idea and predictions for the future', in Aiken, L.H. (ed.) *Nursing in the 80's: Crises, Opportunities, Challenges*, Philadelphia: J.B. Lippincott.

Haines, J. (1993) 'The nurse practitioner: A discussion paper', Canadian Nurses' Association, Ontario, February.

Henderson, V. (1978) 'The concept of nursing', *Journal of Advanced Nursing*, vol. 3, pp. 113–30.

Iliffe, J. (1994) 'Educating for advanced practice—What do nurse practitioners really need?', Conference Paper, 6th National Nursing Education Conference, 28–30 September.

Jacobs, S. (1998) 'Advanced nursing practice in New Zealand', *Nursing Praxis in New Zealand*, vol. 13, no. 3, pp. 4–12.

Lamp, The (1994a) 'Editorial', vol. 51, no. 5, pp. 4–5.

Lamp, The (1994b) 'Editorial', vol. 51, no. 7, p. 9.

Land, S. (1998) 'Barriers and benefits learned from the American advanced nursing practitioner', Paper, The Nursing Profession and Advanced Nursing Practice AIC Worldwide Conference, Sydney, December.

Morewood-Northrop, M. (1994) 'Nursing in the north west territories', *The Canadian Nurse*, March pp. 26–31.

Napier, R. (1996) 'Branch rejects "flawed" nurse practitioner report', *The NSW Doctor*, May, p. 24.

Nelson, B. (1992) '"Independent nurse practitioners"—The AMA perspective', NSW Nurses' Association Annual Conference Professional Day, Sydney.

NSW Department of Health (1993) *Nurse Practitioner Review Stage 2*, vols 1 & 11, June.

NSW Department of Health (1995) *Nurse Practitioner Project Stage 3: Final Report of the Steering Committee*, unpublished.

NSW Nurse Practitioner Project (1995) *Pilot Project Reports to the NSW Department of Health*, unpublished.

Registered Nurses Association of Ontario (1997) 'Registered nurses welcome third reading of nurse practitioner legislation', *www.rnao.org/mr ar22.htm*

Sackett, D.L. (1974) 'The Burlington randomized trial of the nurse practitioner: Health outcomes of patients', *Annals of Internal Medicine*, vol. 80, no. 2, pp. 137–42.

Safriet, B.J. (1992) 'Health care dollars and regulatory sense: The role of advanced practice nursing', *Yale Journal of Regulation*, vol. 9, no. 2, pp. 417–87.

Spitzer, W.O., Sackett, D.L., Sibley, J.C., Roberts, R.S., Gent, M., Kergin, D.J., Hackett, B.C. and Olynich, A. (1974) 'The Burlington randomized trial of the nurse practitioner', *The New England Journal of Medicine*, vol. 290, no. 5, pp. 251–6.

Van Der Horst, M.L. (1992) 'Canada's health care system provides lessons for NPs', *Nurse Practitioner*, vol. 17, no. 8, pp. 44–58.

Waller, S. (1998) 'The UKCC's work on nurse practitioners and clinical nurse specialists', *Emergency Nurse*, vol. 6, no. 3, pp. 12–14.

4 The NSW Nurse Practitioner Project

Amanda Adrian & Jane O'Connell

INTRODUCTION

> The development of the nurse practitioner (and its equivalent) role in the US has been a very much more 'back door approach'. We have yet to openly debate, at a system and health policy level, the endorsement of their role as legitimate providers of quality health services. While this has not happened, this very important role remains vulnerable (Professor Donna Diers, Yale University School of Nursing).

This is a precis of a statement made by Professor Donna Diers at a forum in 1994 held for the NSW Nurse Practitioner Project. Professor Diers' remarks were made when commenting on the differences between the evolution of nurse practitioners in the United States and Australia. They were particularly directed at the lengthy consultative approach being taken by the NSW Department of Health in considering the legitimisation of the role of nurse practitioners in New South Wales, an initiative that had commenced four years previously at the 1990 NSW Nurses' Association's Annual Conference. This conference was a major landmark in the history of the nursing profession in Australia. In a huge auditorium filled with nurses at the Professional Day of the Conference the NSW Nurse Practitioner Project was effectively launched when the then NSW Minister for Health, was issued with a challenge by a nurse asking what seemed an innocent enough question from the audience. The Minister was requested to explore the issue of nurse practitioners being bona fide, rather than de facto, providers of health care—a challenge he accepted.

So began a formal eight-year process that has tested the professional tolerance and political nerve of the nursing profession, the health bureaucracy and the state and federal governments of the time. Over the years 1990–98, a number of discrete stages in the formal process can be identified.

STAGE 1

Stage 1 was a two-year, two-part process. The first part began with a Task Force chaired by the NSW Chief Nursing Officer to plan what to do. The second part involved a Working Party of representatives from key nursing organisations in New South Wales. Their role was first to review a joint submission made to the Task Force by the NSW Nurses' Association and the NSW College of Nursing, two of the peak nursing organisations, representing industrial and professional interests. The second element of this group's commission was to prepare a Discussion Paper.

Subsequently in June 1992, the NSW Minister for Health released the Discussion Paper. It was titled 'The Role and Function of Nurse Practitioners in New South Wales', and was circulated widely 'for the purpose of stimulating debate amongst health professionals, health care providers, consumers and government organisations' (NSW Department of Health 1993, p. 1/1). Stimulate debate, it certainly did! The receipt of approximately 300 written responses to the NSW Department of Health followed significant media coverage:

> Respondents included medical organisations, nursing organisations, Area and Regional Health Services, hospitals, other health care groups, tertiary education institutions, government departments and consumer groups. While a number of individual health professionals submitted responses, there was only a limited response from consumer groups. *The submissions clearly revealed a polarisation of opinion on the attitudes and arguments expressed in the Discussion Paper* [authors' emphasis] (NSW Department of Health 1993, p. 1/1).

STAGE 2

A second Working Party with much broader representation of stakeholders including medical and nursing professional organisations, health department, health management and consumer groups was convened in March 1993, chaired by an independent person. While the deliberations of this group were confidential, most of the members have described the process as both difficult and confronting. The then Branch Secretary of the Australian Medical Association (AMA) (NSW Branch) described it thus: 'The working party's deliberations were arduous, tense and at times bitter' (Nicholson 1993, p. 9).

There were three Terms of Reference for the Working Party (NSW Department of Health 1993, p. 1/2):

- to analyse the submissions and comments on the Discussion Paper, as circulated
- to discuss issues arising from the Discussion Paper and the analyses of the comments
- to develop the final report, making recommendations for consideration by the Minister for Health.

Central to the 15 recommendations made in the review was that a series of pilot projects be set up to scientifically evaluate the role of nurse practitioners in different Australian settings (NSW Department of Health 1993, p. 0/7). This recommendation flowed from the Working Party's recognition of the paucity of literature on the real and potential role for nurse practitioners in Australia, although the anecdotes abounded. It was agreed that the proposed pilot studies would allow assessment of the community and professional reactions to the role of nurse practitioners, and provide the opportunity to examine the role in terms of feasibility, safety, effectiveness, quality and cost under the auspices of a multi-disciplinary evaluation committee (NSW Department of Health 1993, p. 3/7).

As a result of the difficulties with the working party agreeing on a more specific definition, nurse practitioners were defined for the purposes of this Project as: '. . . registered nurses educated for advanced practice, the characteristics of which would be determined by the context in which they practice' (NSW Department of Health 1993, p. 3/5). Interestingly, this broad definition has continued to be used beyond the Nurse Practitioner Project because of its capacity to embrace the extraordinarily diverse range of practice settings and contexts in which a nurse practitioner may work.

It was recommended that at least three pilot sites be established in each of three agreed practice contexts—remote areas, general medical practices, and Area/District Health Services.[1] The areas of practice that could be included in the third context, Area/District Health Services, were limited to sexual health, mental health, outreach services to homeless persons, hospital based emergency departments or units and hospital based maternity services. The other two context categories were not limited in any way. Midwives working in private practice, nurses working in diabetes and asthma care, nurses working in palliative care and nurses working in women's health were not included. While these were areas where it can be argued that nurses have been working autonomously, bringing advanced knowledge, experience and skills to their practice, they appear to have been 'no go' areas.

STAGE 3

In September 1993, the Minister for Health endorsed all of the recommendations and thus began Stage 3 of this increasingly complex, drawn out Project. An independent Chairperson for the Stage 3 Steering Committee was selected, a Project Manager was employed to manage the over-all Project and the Steering Committee was convened. In addition to a number of stalwarts from Stage 2, a number of new members joined the team. Some of the new blood came from the same organisations that were represented during Stage 2, while others represented organisations added to the Steering Committee for Stage 3 of the Project. The appointment of two people from the then Commonwealth Department of Human Services and Health indicated the expanding interest that this Project was generating outside the state's boundaries.

In mid January 1994, an Expression of Interest (EOI) was published widely across Australia in the national, New South Wales state and local press, as well as in key nursing and medical publications. The EOI was designed to begin the process of informing the professions and the community about the pilot projects, as well as to seek proposals from interested parties to become pilot research sites for Stage 3. Enormous interest was generated.

In June 1994 the Minister for Health announced that the ten recommended pilot sites were to be funded. These ten sites were:

- Wilcannia Hospital primary and emergency care service
- Wagga Wagga Base Hospital emergency and primary care service
- Urana Multi-Purpose Service/McCaughey Memorial Hospital primary and emergency care service (also a pilot site for a Multi Purpose Services, a joint Commonwealth and state initiative)
- Wallsend Primary Care Service, a GP run primary care service located in the Hunter Valley
- Kable Street GP Practice, a GP practice in Windsor, where the focus was to be on aged care

- Hunter GP Practices, two GP practices located in small mining communities in the Hunter Valley, where the focus was on women's health
- Shoalhaven Memorial Hospital, Nowra, a hospital maternity service
- Kirketon Road Centre, primary health care, outreach services, sexual health service for homeless youth and sex workers at Kings Cross
- Matthew Talbot Hostel for Homeless Men nursing service— a non-government organisation located in Woolloomooloo
- Concord Hospital and Royal Prince Alfred Hospitals' emergency and primary care services, which formed a combined pilot site, and probably the most controversial of the pilot sites.

While nine of the chosen sites provided what can be described generically as 'primary care services', there was immense diversity across the pilot sites chosen.

The negotiations to develop appropriate competencies and clinical guidelines or protocols in each of the pilot sites were difficult for a number of reasons. Lack of resources (human and financial) and sensitivities related to professional boundaries were two primary barriers. Each pilot project team was required to oversee their development and endorse the clinical guidelines, protocols and competencies. With a multi-disciplinary team, that was not always plain sailing. Ten new partnerships had to be built within a very short period, with all the inherent pain and negotiation.

The next step for the Steering Committee was to reach agreement that the clinical guidelines or protocols and competencies met their requirements. This was also a difficult process given the diversity of interests reflected by the stake holder members.

It was always intended that each of the pilot sites would have a research study that could stand alone, as well as form part of the broader Nurse Practitioner Project. Many of the sites made the most of this opportunity to explore the role and its benefits for their communities. The Project was not trying to prove that nurses were good doctors. Indeed, the emphasis with each of the pilot projects was to highlight what it is that nurses do. However, there are clearly overlaps. An editorial in a local nursing publication highlighted the issues:

> No duty 'belongs' to anyone. There is very little restriction placed on a nurse's practice by legislation. Most restrictions come from custom and practice. Traditionally, members of the health care team share the provision of similar services depending upon the environment in

which the service is provided and who is the most appropriate person to provide the service in that environment. This blurring of roles occurs in all areas of living—you can buy meat at the butcher, but also at the supermarket; you can buy vitamins at the pharmacy, but also at the health food store and the supermarket. New concepts pose new challenges and should not be measured against old and tired dogma. Life is characterised by progress and an examination of the role of nurse practitioners embraces progress (*The Lamp* 1994).

The recommendations of the *Nurse Practitioner Project Stage 3: Final Report of the Steering Committee* flowed from the rigorous, scientific analysis of the data that were collected as part of the pilot research sites. The Report's findings were unequivocal:

> The evidence from the research conducted by each of the pilot projects and the across-project research supports that nurse practitioners are feasible, safe and effective in their roles and provide quality health services in the range of settings researched.
> The strong evidence emerging from these pilot projects shows that in the areas of the research studies, the role of the nurse practitioner was a feasible one which variously had: added value to already existing health services; provided a new and valuable additional service; or provided the only available service. The safety of the role was established in as much as nurse practitioners satisfactorily followed protocols/clinical guidelines in 96% of cases[2] and their clinical decisions and management were judged to be reasonable, supported by the evidence from clinical review.
> The research points to the conclusions that the nurse practitioner service was also effective in improving access by consumers/patients and satisfying consumer/patient expectations, predominantly achieving interdisciplinary collaboration and in servicing people who would otherwise have fallen outside the boundaries of conventional health care services. Expected standards of quality were also achieved during the research by a reported high level of professional behaviour, management capability and positive consumer reports. Economic evaluation and examination of outcomes, while lesser components of the research methodology because of limitations set by the context of Stage 3, also lend support to these findings.
> . . . valuable empirical evidence provided by the ten (10) pilot project sites (a sample size of 2706 interludes of care were examined), together with the outcomes of discussions on issues brought forward from Stage 2, assured the majority of the members of the Steering Committee of the potential positive contribution to be made by establishing the nurse practitioner role within the NSW health care system (NSW Department of Health 1995, pp. i–iii).[3]

As well as the research component, the recommendations in the Report reflected the extensive range of issues that were grappled with over the three stages of the Project to the end of 1995.

The recommendations ranged across matters of legitimisation, edu-

cation, accreditation, clinical assessment (including ordering investigations), clinical management (including prescribing medications and
referrals), funding and professional indemnity. However, the recommendations also addressed a number of other areas that relate to the
provision of services by nurse practitioners, improving communication
and building better relationships with both health care consumers and
(particularly) other health service providers.

Much myth and legend still prevail about the existing roles and
potential roles of nurse practitioners. The manifestations of these
concerns are evident in some of the safeguards that were negotiated in
the recommendations by the non nursing members of the Steering
Committee. It is interesting and not surprising that it is these particular
recommendations that were most criticised by members of the nursing
profession. The recommendations related to the identification of a local
agreed need and the recommendations regarding referral were those
that have attracted the most criticism.

Not to be forgotten is that the Steering Committee was made up
of a number of diverse key stakeholders, all of whom were identified as
having significant 'interests' in the legitimisation of nurse practitioners
as bone fide providers of health services in New South Wales. The
debate around the committee table was fierce and at times very difficult.
While the recommendations may not have been totally palatable to
all nurses and did not always reflect the views and position of the
nursing organisations represented on the Steering Committee, they
were the product of the cut and thrust of this process of negotiation.
They also indicate the considerable compromises that most members
of the Committee had to make in the interests of achieving a way
forward.

On reflection, the potency of the emotions evident in the debate
was not surprising. The players included nurses who believed passion-
ately that the role of nurse practitioners should be recognised. Central
also were the consumers who were vitally concerned about ensuring
that any health service provider is adequately skilled, educated and
experienced to provide the needed services. This group was also ada-
mant that safeguards were available to protect consumers, and insisted
processes were in place to ensure the services met consumer needs, not
just service provider's wishes. Then there were the representatives of
the medical profession. One only has to read the Report from Stage 2
of the Project to realise that there was considerable opposition to the
notion of nurse practitioners from powerful factions within the medical
profession, particularly those representing industrial interests. This has
not changed in the main, although several key medical organisations

have stated their support for the position negotiated, with all the safe-guards in place. These have primarily been professional organisations.

Other interesting features highlighted by the research and the Steering Committee negotiations were, first, the general lack of under-standing and ambivalence in the community about nurse prac-titioners. Second, there was an absolute prohibition on the opening up of the Commonwealth Medicare provider payment system to nurses.

A FRAMEWORK FOR IMPLEMENTATION

The risk with such a controversial Project and outcome was that it could end up in limbo. Certainly great effort was expended in attempt-ing to ensure its relegation to that domain. Realistically, viewing the situation after Stage 3, there were two options. First, to accept the negotiated position of the multi-disciplinary Steering Committee with all its safeguards and notions of partnerships and collaboration. Or alternatively, to create an environment where the bunker positions are retreated to and the skirmishing continued while the role of the nurse practitioner developed in an unstructured way and the devices used to cover up the accountabilities of clinical decision making are perpetuated. These artificial devices include 'standing orders', 'emer-gency telephone orders', special mechanisms to enable for remote area nursing practice that are politically (not practically) unacceptable in urban settings, as well as other activities to circumvent current legislation or health service policy. These are familiar ruses used widely in the health system.

Despite the cynicism of many nurses who believed that the Project had stalled after Stage 3, significant efforts were made by a number of key organisations and individuals in the nursing profession to ensure that this did not happen. Much negotiation continued, while at the same time the NSW Department of Health was earnest in its endeavours to develop the means by which the recommendations could be implemented after the Minister for Health supported this position in February 1997.

The focus of the activity was to identify and prioritise action in the areas of:

* legislative amendments required
* the process and criteria for the accreditation of nurse practitioners
* refining the principles for the development of clinical guidelines

- the policy for the establishment of nurse practitioner services (NSW Department of Health 1998).

The *Framework for the Implementation of Nurse Practitioner Services in NSW* was released by the Director-General for Health in August 1998 and outlined the policy and legislative changes that were to occur. Subsequent to that, and despite a significant, and by now, predictable media campaign by several key medical associations, the *Nurses Amendment (Nurse Practitioners) Act* was passed by both houses of the New South Wales Parliament with minimal debate and no amendments in September and October of that same year. Assent was given on 2 November 1998.

Legislative amendments

The legislative amendments highlight the significant achievements of this long and torrid Project. They are testament to the tenacity of many clinging to a vision based on the recognition of the health care needs of different populations. The new provisions are also a major point in the 'coming of age' of the nursing profession and its acceptance of a notable mantle of clinical accountability.

The *Nurses Amendment (Nurse Practitioners) Act 1998* (NSW) has as the object of the Act to amend the *Nurses Act 1991*:

- to allow the Nurses Registration Board to authorise certain registered nurses to practise as nurse practitioners; and
- to allow the Director-General of the Department of Health to approve guidelines relating to the functions of nurse practitioners, and to allow such guidelines to make provision for the possession, use, supply and prescription of certain substances by nurse practitioners; and
- to prevent an unauthorised person from using the title 'nurse practitioner' or otherwise holding himself or herself out to be a nurse practitioner.

The Act also amends the *Poisons and Therapeutic Goods Act 1966* to allow the Director-General of the Department of Health to authorise a nurse practitioner to possess, use, supply or prescribe substances specified in the Poisons List (other than drugs of addiction) in accordance with the guidelines approved by the Director-General (NSW Parliament 1998, p. 1).

Amendments to the Nurses Act 1991 (NSW)

Application, determination, authorisation and certification. The Act enables a registered nurse to make an application to the NSW Nurses' Registration Board for authorisation to practise as a nurse practitioner. If the application is granted, a certificate of authorisation to practise as a nurse practitioner is issued and the details of authorisation are entered in the Register of Nurses. Provisions are made for temporary authorisation in certain circumstances, and a registered nurse that has their application refused may appeal against the determination.

Board functions. The Act supplements the functions of the NSW Nurses' Registration Board to give it similar functions to those already present in the Nurses Act in relation to authorised midwives, such as being capable of imposing requirements or conditions relating to their practice. It also allows the Board to recognise different areas of practice as a nurse practitioner. The latter function will undoubtedly relate to the different areas of clinical practice, such as mental health care, the different arenas of primary care, midwifery and palliative care.

Clinical guidelines for clinical assessment and management. The Act requires the Director-General of the NSW Department of Health to approve guidelines relating to the clinical assessment, management and follow-up practices of nurse practitioners. Any contravention of the approved guidelines by a nurse practitioner may constitute professional misconduct or unsatisfactory professional conduct.

Prohibition on 'holding out'. The Act makes it an offence for someone who is not an authorised nurse practitioner to claim to be, or hold themselves out to be, a nurse practitioner.

Power to make regulations. Amendments to the Act enable regulations to be made relating to nurse practitioners, including those that provide for the regulation and supervision of the practice of nurse practitioners.

Other amendments. Further amendments to the Act include: general requirements for authorisation to practise as a nurse practitioner, and are the same as those that apply to registration as a nurse generally; provisions that provide for the suspension and cancellation of authorisation to practise as a nurse practitioner; and amendments to provide for evidentiary matters in relation to authorisation to practise as a nurse practitioner.

Amendments to the Poisons and Therapeutic Goods Act 1966 (NSW)

The Act allows the Director-General of the NSW Department of Health to authorise a nurse practitioner or a class of nurse practitioners to possess, use, supply or prescribe any poison or restricted substance, except for drugs of addiction.

This is the first time that nurses have had the capacity to do this in a manner that directly recognises the nurse (in this case, an authorised nurse practitioner) as possessor, user, supplier or prescriber in legislation. Nurses have been bestowed with secondary rights in the past but these were shrouded in the devices of 'standing orders', '24-hour telephone orders' and other such means.

The authorisation may only be given if the Director-General approves the guidelines relating to nurse practitioners outlined in Section 78A of the Nurses Act and those guidelines provide for the use, supply or prescription by nurse practitioners of substances specified in the Poisons List.

A nurse practitioner authorised by the Director-General in this way is exempted from the following offences:

- the offence of supplying the substance otherwise than by wholesale;
- the offence of having the substance in their possession;
- the offence of hawking of the substance.

In addition, a person who supplies a poison or restricted substance on the prescription of a nurse practitioner, obtains possession of the substance in accordance with the prescription of a nurse practitioner, or has possession of a substance for the purpose of delivering it to a nurse practitioner, is exempted from the relevant offences under the Act.

Amendments to the Act also make it an offence to:

- obtain a restricted substance from a nurse practitioner by means of a false or misleading representation;
- forge or fraudulently alter a prescription of a nurse practitioner;
- obtain a prescription for a restricted substance from a nurse practitioner by means of false or misleading representation.

Authorisation of nurse practitioners

Under the Act, registered nurses wishing to be authorised as nurse practitioners will have to meet quite stringent requirements of education, experience and demonstrated skills in the context of practice in which authorisation is sought before they are eligible to be entered onto the professional register as nurse practitioners. Only then will they acquire certain exclusive rights such as those relating to naming (holding themselves out as nurse practitioners) and prescribing. Nurse practitioners are highly skilled, experienced, expert nurses, *not* beginning or novice nurses.

The authorisation of nurse practitioners does not mean that there will be the development of another level of nurses. What it does mean is that registered nurses who have developed higher level skills in certain areas of practice that are complemented by appropriate education and experience in the area of practice, may seek authorisation.

The *Framework* document (NSW Department of Health 1998) sets out 'Guidelines for the Process of Authorisation of Nurse Practitioners in NSW'. The key issues, not highlighted or detailed in the legislation are:

- a Nurse Practitioner Authorisation Committee is to be established by the NSW Nurses' Registration Board with the key professional stakeholder composition outlined in Recommendation 3.2.4 of the *Nurse Practitioner Project Stage 3: Final Report of the Steering Committee*
- recognition for the authorisation as a nurse practitioner and their context of practice is to be noted on the Authority to Practice
- the NSW Nurses' Registration Board Authorisation Committee will review the applicant's demonstrated experience against the essential criteria for authorisation, specific to the context of practice
- Authorisation as a nurse practitioner in a specific context of practice will be granted for a three year period after which re-authorisation will be necessary (NSW Department of Health 1998, pp. 1–2).

The criteria for authorisation as a nurse practitioner in New South Wales include:

- a registered nurse on List A in New South Wales
- relevant post registration qualifications or equivalent, enabling expert practice in the context in which accreditation is sought
- demonstration of 5000 hours of current practice in an advanced practice role, articulating competency standards for an advanced nurse clinician, as well as specialty standards in the context in which authorisation is sought
- demonstrated skills and knowledge associated with the identified

privileges relevant to the context of practice, including pharmacology and clinical assessment

- demonstrated ongoing professional development, that is, attendance and active participation at relevant seminars, workshops and conferences (NSW Department of Health 1998, p. 2).

The Nurse Practitioner Authorisation Committee established by the NSW Nurses Registration Board is charged with further refining the criteria for accreditation of nurse practitioners, including assessment processes and to make recommendations to the Board. Other responsibilities of this Committee will include providing advice on requirements for individuals to achieve authorisation and liaising with relevant specialist nursing associations on issues related to authorisation of nurse practitioners (NSW Department of Health 1998, p. 2).

The *Framework* document further clarifies the position on the professional indemnity for nurse practitioners, making the following points:

- all nurse practitioners working as employees will be covered by their employer through vicarious liability
- there will be an obligation on any nurse practitioners working in the public sector under agreement, contract or in any other arrangement who are not covered by vicarious liability to carry personal indemnity insurance
- the NSW Department of Health recommends that nurse practitioners working outside the public sector who are not covered by vicarious liability have personal indemnity insurance
- the NSW Nurses Registration Board will provide relevant information concerning professional indemnity to all applicants (NSW Department of Health 1998, p. 3).

There are no 'grandparent provisions' for existing registered nurses to gain authorisation without meeting each of the criteria as recommended in the *Stage 3 Report*. Any prospective nurse practitioners will be required to undergo a full assessment against all the authorisation criteria by the Board. No special interim arrangements will be made to enable a registered nurse a period of grace to 'catch up'.

The legislative and policy framework for nurse practitioners working in New South Wales is based on them working with guidelines relating to the clinical assessment, management and follow-up relevant to their context of practice. This requirement is seen by some as draconian and effectively limiting the autonomy of the nurse practitioner to make decisions based on their clinical judgement. However, this step of requiring the development of practice guidelines to provide a framework for a nurse practitioner's clinical practice is not out of line with the 'evidence based practice' movement gaining increasing acceptance by health clinicians generally. Clinical practice guidelines are to be developed based on the best scientific evidence available. In Australia the National Health and Medical Research Council (NH&MRC) have developed *Guidelines for the Development and Implementation of Clinical Practice Guidelines* (NH&MRC 1995). These Guidelines have been used to create a set of principles that will guide health services in the development, by a multi-disciplinary team at a local level, of their own context and service specific clinical guidelines for nurse practitioners. The principles outline the importance of consultation with relevant professional organisations and the process for approval. The original guidelines were revised in 1999 and have been reissued as the *Guide to the Development, Implementation and Evaluation of Clinical Practice Guidelines* (NH&MRC 1999).

Developed by the multi-disciplinary team (including relevant representation from the medical, nursing, pharmacy and allied health professions), clinical guidelines will address specific clinical presentations and guide the nurse practitioner in clinical assessment, clinical management and evaluation. Any formulary developed as part of the clinical guidelines will require approval by the Director-General of the NSW Department of Health for nurse practitioners to be authorised to possess, use, supply and prescribe under the *Poisons and Therapeutic Goods Act 1966* (NSW). The Director-General will not give approval unless the local group developing the clinical guidelines demonstrates that the requisite steps have been followed.

The NSW Department of Health identified a strategic though narrow plan for the introduction of authorised nurse practitioners in New South Wales. Continuing to sustain vocal criticism from several groups within the medical profession it is hoped that the plan will allay the fears and demonstrate that a safe collaborative model of health service delivery involving nurse practitioners is possible.

In the first instance public, rural Area Health Services and the Corrections Health Service have been requested to identify areas of need and, following agreement with the Department, Areas will be responsible to ensure that the process outlined in the framework is followed. It is the responsibility of Area Health Services, in consultation with key stakeholders including general practitioners, to plan services responsive to the interests of the local community and within available resources. On receipt of detailed submissions from Area

Health Services, the Department will consult with relevant groups before final approval is given for any nurse practitioner position.

The New South Wales nurse practitioner model does not include access to provider numbers. This was a matter that was non-negotiable during the Project and, indeed, many nurses felt that pursuing that funding model may prove counter-productive for nursing services and that other more innovative funding models should be explored.

It was envisaged that due to the legislative changes required and the development of the accreditation processes there would be a substantial lead-time of at least 12 to 18 months before authorised nurse practitioners would be employed in the New South Wales health system.

The Director-General has arranged that a state-wide committee including representatives of the Royal Australian College of General Practitioners (NSW), the NSW College of Nursing, NSW Nurses' Association and the Australian Medical Association (NSW) will oversee the implementation and evaluation of the *Framework*.

CONCLUSION

The success of this laborious and difficult process with all its political and professional fallout will only become evident over time. Whether a negotiated process such as this—with the delivery of what is comparable to a healthy newborn baby that needs time to develop and mature—is preferable to a more organic and perhaps less predictable process of evolution is, as yet, unclear.

ENDNOTES

1   In 1993–97 the rural health areas of New South Wales were divided into District Health Services. Since 1997, many of these have merged to create larger Health Services administered in a similar way to the metropolitan Area Health Services.

2   In approximately half of the 4% of cases where protocols/clinical guidelines were not followed the deviations were deemed justified by a multi-disciplinary clinical review team. (Assessment: deviation justified 1.6%; deviation not justified 1.1%; missing data 1.3%. Management: deviation justified 2.0%; deviation not justified 1.6%; missing data 0.4%.)

3   The AMA (NSW Branch) subsequently notified the NSW Department of Health of their dissenting position in relation to the recommendations and the Report.

REFERENCES

Lamp, The (1994) 'Editorial', vol. 51, no. 7, pp. 9–11.

National Health and Medical Research Council (NH&MRC) (1995) Guidelines for the Development of Clinical Practice Guidelines, 1st edn, Canberra: AGPS, October.

NH&MRC (1999) Guide to the Development, Implementation and Evaluation of Clinical Practice Guidelines, Canberra: AGPS.

NSW Department of Health (1993) Nurse Practitioner Review Stage 2, vols 1 & 11, June.

NSW Department of Health (1995) Nurse Practitioner Project Stage 3: Final Report of the Steering Committee, published report.

NSW Department of Health (1998) Framework for the Implementation of Nurse Practitioner Services in NSW, State Health Publication (NB) 970106, August.

NSW Parliament (1998) Nurses Amendment (Nurse Practitioners) Bill 1998, Explanatory Note.

Nicholson, M. (1993) 'Plan keeps nurse practitioners in check', NSW Doctor, October.

COMMENTARY—CHAPTERS 3 AND 4

Chris Murphy

Amanda Adrian and Jane O'Connell present a clear and concise view of global trends which have influenced the development of the nurse practitioner role worldwide. In the United Kingdom, it was the demand for improved health care, an emphasis on chronic illness and trends towards preventive approaches to health care, which led the way for incentives to change and expand on the role of the practice nurse to one of nurse practitioner in primary health care.

The *Framework for the Implementation of Nurse Practitioner Services in NSW* recognises the importance of professional links for consultation and review between nurse practitioners and nominated medical practitioners. It is clearly recognised that collaboration between health professionals is fundamental to the quality of health services. In my view this is central to the facilitation of partnerships in health care.

An important aspect of the development of the nurse practitioner role is recognition of that role. In the United Kingdom, there was no formal policy or regulatory framework, leading to confusion about the nurse practitioner role for consumers and health professionals alike. The development of specialised programs for nurse practitioner education was not formalised, leading to further confusion. Australian nurses should be commended for approaching the implementation of the nurse practitioner role in such a rigorous way.

However, acceptance of the role of the nurse practioner in primary health care by GP colleagues may be more difficult here in Australia than in the United Kingdom. One of the main barriers may be that the concept of the primary health care team is not familiar to many GPs. Few will have had prior experience of working with nurses in general practice. There may be a limited understanding of the potential role of the nurse in the provision of primary health care services within the context of a multi-disciplinary team.

Many GPs currently work in isolation from their medical

peers, some are working in direct competition with their peers. The introduction of a nurse practitioner may be seen as a threat rather than a potential complement to the delivery of primary health care services.

One solution might be the provision of funding so that GPs may be directly reimbursed for nurse practitioner services. This would facilitate the acceptance of the role, involve GPs directly in the development of the role, therefore fostering the development of trust and mutual understanding of the potential of nurse practitioners to complement existing care.

Future directions include a shift from the traditional role of tending the sick and carrying out doctors' orders, to one of diagnosis and treatment. These changes in role imply greater authority and power within health care systems but may also bring conflict with GPs. Professional communication, joint education and clear role definition would assist role analysis and help in the resolution of potential conflicts.

PART II

Influence on practice

5   Suicide

Pierre Baume

INTRODUCTION

If suicide rates are maintained at current levels, over 60 000 Australians will have lost their lives by suicide in the next 20 years (ABS 1998). Like many western nations, Australia has not been exempt from this tragedy, a tragedy made more poignant with a substantial increase in rates being observed in younger generations. This increase in rates of suicide among young people in the 1990s has been emerging as a major public health concern since the early 1960s. It has, however, not received much attention by policy makers until the beginning of this decade.

Suicide is a tragic loss of human life, which has profound personal effects for those closely associated with the death. There are many unanswered questions about suicide and a multitude of conflicting theories concerning the roles played by mental illness and social factors, as well as the existence and nature of predisposing factors, and the parallel issues of proper and effective prevention (Beck et al. 1993; Diekstra & Garnefski 1995; Freud 1964; Hassan 1995; Lester 1992a). There is never one reason why a person may choose to end their life as reasons are always multiple. How to best prevent suicide is therefore both complex and obvious. Trying to identify the chain of causal and/or triggering factors may be highly individual. Deriving an overall understanding and developing effective strategies, therefore, is perhaps one of the most complex and challenging problems faced by nurses today.

Suicides represent premature and often preventable deaths. This provides a great opportunity for prevention and intervention. The majority of suicidal individuals inform others of their intention to kill themselves beforehand, whether these are friends, relatives or health care professionals (Baume, McTaggart & Cantor 1997). Many suicidal individuals tend to remain ambivalent about whether or not they should kill themselves right to the very end. Suicide demands that everybody concerned with clinical care, especially in non psychiatric environments, should be clear about both their own attitudes to suicide and the procedures to be adopted in managing individuals at risk.

This chapter focuses on suicidal behaviour and its associated risk factors. Although suicide occurs across the life span the greatest emphasis in this chapter revolves around the self-destructive behaviour of young people. An introduction into the scope of the problem, theoretical models to understand its meaning and the factors that may be associated with suicide and attempted suicide are discussed. This chapter also attempts to explore the health and social issues associated with suicide and identifies a number of the most pertinent factors associated with suicidal behaviour. Risk factors can be identified and used in any setting as a foundation to inform nursing practice in the care of those individuals with suicidal behaviour.

DEFINING SUICIDE

The definition of suicide and suicidal behaviours has been the subject of considerable debate. Indeed, suicidal behaviours can be defined as the intention or self-infliction of injury or death. Although many behaviours fall within the broad spectrum of this definition of suicide, intentional risk or self-harm, such as chronic substance abuse, habitual risk (e.g. driving over the speed limit, smoking, binge drinking) willful self-neglect and non-compliance with the treatment of serious physical illness, may require a wider interpretation. The degree to which such behaviours share a common basis with suicide in cause and treatment is still controversial.

In this chapter, the element of intention has been considered a key defining characteristic of suicide, while related self-destructive behaviours have been seen as somewhat less intentional and selfconcious in origin.

The term suicide emerged with the birth of science and the secular world of the mid-1600s (Shneidman 1969). Over the centuries suicide has been perceived differently in many cultures. Islam, Judaism and Christianity condemn it with suicide attempts in many of those cultures still punishable by laws. In Australia, it wasn't until the 1970s that the act of suicide was decriminalised, while the act of attempted suicide still remained a crime in most states until the early 1990s (Hallenstein 1994).

At times, some cultures have encouraged the act. The Brahmans of India tolerated suicide and the voluntary suicide of an Indian widow (suttee) was highly praised, while in ancient Greece and Rome convicted criminals were permitted to take their own lives (Fedden 1980). In Asia, Hara Kiri or self-disembowelment, a Japanese custom, was long practised as a ceremonial right. Samurais were granted the privilege of punishing themselves in this way for wrongdoing to escape the humiliation of failure or to shame ones enemy (Hassan 1995).

Our current understanding of suicide and self-destructive behaviours, however, reflects a psychoanalytic and sociological tradition developed towards the end of the last century. Durkheim (1951) in 'Le suicide' provided the first population based statistical study of suicide in 1897. He postulated that suicide rates were usually predictable in terms of social factors that influence them. More recently suicide has been described as a drama in the mind or 'psyche-ache': 'a conscious act of self induced annihilation best understood as a multi-dimensional malaise in the need for the individual who defines an issue for which suicide is perceived as the best solution' (Shneidman 1993, p. 203).

The above discussion prompts two observations. First, attitudes towards the rationality of suicide have clearly changed over time. There is little doubt that some cultures or individuals would consider irrational what others in time may have seen as not only rational, but laudable. Second, there is an obvious connection between the designation of suicide as rational and what is socially acceptable. Although it is not the intention of this chapter to resolve this controversy, these views reflect the difficulty and complexity in defining the nature of suicide.

PREVALENCE

Each year over 2500 deaths in Australia are recorded as suicide and this is probably an under-estimation of the true picture (ABS 1998). Suicide is now the leading cause of death from all external causes for all age groups, ahead of motor vehicle accidents and well ahead of homicides, which have remained relatively constant for the greater part of this century (ABS 1998).

Despite much publicity about increases in overall Australian suicide rates in the media, the overall rates of suicide in Australia were similar at the end of the twentieth century to those at the end of the nineteenth century (see Table 5.1). During the past 100 years or so these rates have been subject to significant fluctuations. Rates peaked in the 1930s depression and were lowest during, and immediately after, the Second World War (see Figure 5.1). A significant increase is noted for both males and females in the late 1950s followed by a decrease for both genders in the early 1970s. These later changes were primarily associated with the increase in barbiturate overdoses, which subsided with the introduction of safer benzodiazepine sedatives. However, since the early 1960s, rates for males have risen again sharply and this rise is mainly associated with the increase in young male suicides (Baume, Cantor & McTaggart 1998).

Table 5.1   Australian rate of suicide: 1887 and 1997 per 100 000 population

Year	Male	Female	Total
1887	20.6	5.5	12.5
1997	23.3	6.2	14.7

Source: ABS 1998

Figure 5.1   Rates of suicide, Australia: Males, females and total, all ages, 1881–1997

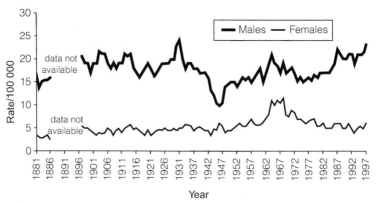

Source: ABS 1998

SUICIDE IN YOUNG PEOPLE

In the past suicide has increased as a function of age, whereby the older the person the greater the risks (Hassan 1995) (see Figure 5.2).

Figure 5.2 Rates of suicide, Australia: By age group, males 1961 and 1997

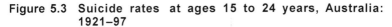

Source: ABS 1998

The rates for people age 65 years and over have nearly halved in the last two decades. Although the rates for those over the age of 75 years remain the highest of those in the 65 years and over age group their numbers are still small when compared with those aged under 40 years (Baume & Snowdon 1999). In the general population, rates of suicide in the younger age group (15 to 24 years) have fluctuated (see Figure 5.3). This is due in part to the small number of deaths in this age group. Nevertheless, significant upward trends have been observed in young males: a trend also observed in many other nations (UNICEF 1996). Until the 1960s the rates for young males were around 10 per 100 000 of the population, except for a decline during and immediately after the war years. Unlike the adult population, increases during the

Figure 5.3 Suicide rates at ages 15 to 24 years, Australia: 1921–97

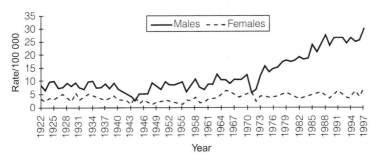

Source: ABS 1998

depression years are not significant in this younger age group. Although rates of suicides for females in the 15 to 24 year age group have remained low for the period 1922 to 1997, their rates have doubled since the 1960s, remaining at around 5 to 7 per 100 000 during the 1980s and 1990s. Suicide rates for 15 to 24 year old males have risen sharply since 1960 from 6.8 per 100 000 to 30.63 per 100 000 in 1997. These suicides now represent 25% of all deaths for males in that age group and 17% of all females. The highest frequency of suicides observed in Australia for males now occurs in those aged 25 to 34 years, or 37.52 per 100 000, and for females, those aged 35 to 44 years or 8.51 per 100 000 (ABS 1998).

COMPARISON BETWEEN STATES AND OTHER COUNTRIES

Available data demonstrate differences between the Australian states and territories over time. The suicide rates for each state and territory for a 32-year period from 1964 to 1995 are provided in Table 5.2. These results demonstrate that Queensland has had rates well above the national average for this 32-year period. Suicide rates always vary between states, but it is notable that Queensland and Tasmania have consistently had rates significantly over the national average, while Victoria and NSW have been below the national average.

Figure 5.4   Deaths by suicide, 15 to 24 years: International data 1991–93

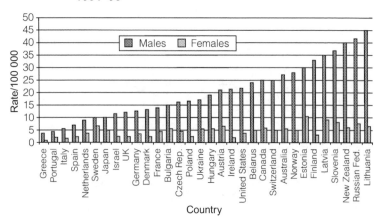

Source: Baume, Cantor & McTaggart 1998

Table 5.2   Suicide rates by state and territory: 1964–95, all ages

	NSW	Vic.	Qld	SA	WA	Tas.	NT	ACT	Total
1964	15.3	10.6	20.1	16.0	15.3	11.5	9.1	10.0	14.6
1965	17.5	11.0	18.1	12.5	13.6	12.0	25.6	11.3	14.8
1966	16.0	10.9	17.0	12.4	15.1	9.2	7.1	10.4	14.0
1967	16.9	13.2	16.8	12.9	13.9	12.8	9.7	8.7	15.0
1968	13.5	11.3	14.1	11.8	12.8	14.0	11.8	8.9	12.7
1969	13.2	10.1	14.6	12.2	11.2	13.3	5.5	14.0	12.2
1970	12.7	11.0	15.2	12.0	11.1	12.9	14.0	9.9	12.4
1971	13.1	14.0	15.1	10.2	14.3	11.8	4.7	7.9	13.3
1972	13.3	11.8	12.4	10.5	12.1	10.7	9.8	5.6	12.2
1973	12.2	9.7	12.8	9.8	11.3	13.6	12.4	9.8	11.3
1974	12.1	10.0	13.3	10.6	10.7	12.8	11.7	8.1	11.4
1975	11.7	9.7	13.9	11.8	7.3	9.8	8.6	8.5	11.0
1976	11.3	8.8	12.1	11.5	10.9	11.2	17.3	10.1	10.7
1977	10.5	11.8	11.5	10.0	11.6	10.1	5.8	12.2	11.0
1978	10.8	9.8	14.5	11.9	10.4	11.7	7.3	9.2	11.1
1979	10.5	11.9	13.4	13.7	9.3	13.3	9.6	8.6	11.6
1980	10.6	11.2	12.1	11.2	10.0	10.6	12.7	5.8	10.9
1981	10.4	10.9	12.8	12.1	10.6	15.2	13.0	9.7	11.2
1982	11.0	11.7	12.3	13.0	12.8	13.7	5.4	7.3	11.7
1983	10.1	12.7	11.2	10.3	10.6	15.9	11.8	11.7	11.2
1984	9.4	11.5	12.4	11.0	12.7	11.7	7.7	13.5	11.0
1985	11.7	10.2	13.3	10.0	12.1	15.8	10.8	11.1	11.6
1986	11.2	12.5	14.7	13.2	11.2	15.5	9.1	12.7	12.4
1987	11.6	15.5	15.7	13.5	13.6	15.1	10.1	15.1	13.8
1988	12.8	12.6	14.9	13.1	13.5	16.0	17.6	11.4	13.3
1989	11.8	11.6	14.5	14.2	11.7	13.0	14.9	12.7	12.5
1990	11.6	11.4	14.6	14.9	13.3	15.1	18.3	12.4	12.7
1991	13.0	13.7	14.3	16.0	12.9	14.4	11.5	11.8	13.6
1992	12.3	12.5	14.1	14.6	12.9	20.4	13.7	10.5	13.1
1993	11.7	11.1	11.8	11.3	12.9	17.6	13.0	9.0	11.8
1994	12.9	11.4	14.2	11.5	12.8	14.8	11.1	12.0	12.7
1995	12.5	12.6	15.1	13.6	12.6	14.0	13.2	11.2	13.1

Source: Baume, Cantor & McTaggart 1998

Although the increasing trend of suicide in young people is worldwide in the 15 to 24 year old age group (Baume 1988, 1995; Diekstra & Garnefski 1995), the high rates when compared to the middle and older age groups seem to be peculiar to Australia and New Zealand. In other western nations the increased rates are usually associated with advancing age (Pritchard 1992). While Australia does not have the highest rate of suicide in young people (see Figure 5.4) it is significant that New Zealand has higher rates. It is also interesting to note that the Japanese and UK rates for young men are less than half of those of Australia.

CULTURAL FACTORS AND METHODS USED FOR SUICIDE

The suicide rate for the Australian indigenous population appears to be substantially higher than in the non-indigenous population, yet until recently suicide was considered uncommon in indigenous communities (Hunter 1993). Research reveals that the rate of suicide in young Aboriginal Australians is as high as 120 per 100 000 or three times higher than the non-indigenous population. This is, however, limited to younger age groups and does not appear to be the case for older Aborigines where the number is extremely low, partly because relatively few indigenous people live to old age (Baume, Cantor & McTaggart 1998).

Migrants under the age of 65 years living in Australia appear to have similar or lower rates of suicide when compared to Australian-born people, although significantly higher rates have been observed among specific elderly migrant populations. This trend applies not just to those countries of birth with traditionally high rates of suicide, for example, Eastern Europe and parts of Asia, but also to certain countries of birth with low rates, for example, Southern Europe, Middle East/Egypt and North-east Asia (Burvill 1998). There are also some clear differences in the selection of suicide methods used by some migrant groups. For example, while overdoses are documented as the main method used by females in Australia, for females from Southern Europe and South-east and North-east Asia, hanging is the most common form. With males, hanging is also a common method for people from Southern and Eastern Europe, former USSR and the Baltic States, Middle East/Egypt, and South-east and North Asia. A comparison of rates and methods among migrant populations in Australia with rates and methods in the country of origin suggest that the socio-cultural factors that migrants bring with them may be important determinants for suicidal behaviour (McDonald & Steel 1997).

There are four major methods used in Australia by both genders: hanging, carbon monoxide poisoning, firearms and ingestion of substances. These account for about 90% of all suicides (see Figures 5.5 and 5.6). Additionally there are other suicides by jumping, lying in front of moving vehicles, drowning, self-burning and the use of a vehicle, but these are far less common in Australia (Cantor & Baume 1998).

A number of important changes in methods of suicide have recently occurred. On the positive side, deaths by drug overdose, after a peak in the 1960s for males and females (primarily due to barbituates), have declined. Much of this reduction has been associ-

Figure 5.5 Rates of suicide, Australia: Males all ages, 1974–97

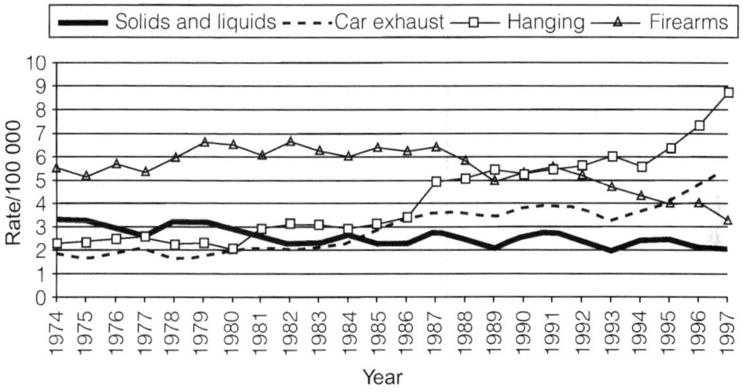

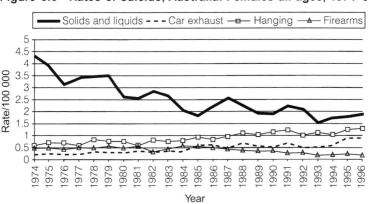

Source: Baume, Cantor & McTaggart 1998

ated with a change in prescribing and resuscitation practices. Nonetheless, self-poisoning, either in terms of attempts or completed suicides, continue to be of concern. It is clear that this method is an important cause of hospitalisation as well as death in both women and men. A rise in deaths from specific substances has also been noted, particularly under the categories of tranquilisers and analgesics (Buckley et al. 1995a, 1995b). In terms of analgesics, while paracetamol continues to top the list and is usually associated with very serious liver damage, even if death does not occur (Jones et al. 1997), it is

Figure 5.6 Rates of suicide, Australia: Females all ages, 1974–97

Source: Baume, Cantor & McTaggart 1998

far less frequent a method in Australia than in the United Kingdom (Farmer 1996). Tricyclic anti-depressants, however, represent almost 20% of all overdose suicides (Baume, Cantor & McTaggart 1998). In a recent study of 2799 suicides, which occurred between 1990 and 1995, the authors reported that 46% of tricyclic anti-depressant deaths were from dotheipin, 23% from amitryptiline, 20% from doxepin, and 8% imipramine overdoses. Of note, the newer anti-depressants, moclobemide, fluoxetine, paroxetine and sertraline, when combined, accounted for less than 1% of those deaths (Baume, Cantor & McTaggart 1998).

Among other methods used by both genders, an alarming fourfold increase in hanging has been noted. There has also been a doubling in carbon monoxide (motor vehicle exhaust) suicides along with speculation that the decline in firearms may have resulted in the substitution of other methods. This does not adequately account for the observation that the rise in suicide by hanging and carbon monoxide is much greater than the decline in firearms. The increase in hanging has also been noted in Aboriginal and non-Aboriginal populations and therefore may be suggestive of broader cultural influences. It has been argued that the media coverage of deaths in custody has promoted a symbolic association of suicide with hanging (Baume & Clinton 1997). However, the small numbers associated with changes in female suicides dictate caution as they may represent random fluctuations rather than real changes in self-destructive behaviours.

Differences in the distribution of suicide methods chosen are also significant between the states. In Tasmania a greater proportion (50%) of all suicides are by firearms. Similarly, the male suicide rates in Queensland are associated with above average rates of firearm suicides. Western Australia, on the other hand, showed an elevated rate of suicide by poisoning using motor vehicle exhaust and by hanging. South Australia also had an above average suicide rate for hanging (Cantor, Turrell & Baume 1996). Young people 15 to 24 years of age tend to select methods similar to those in other age groups, which appear to be gender specific and culturally determined. The distribution, however, varies according to their geographical location. There is a tendency, for example, for firearm suicides to be more likely to occur in rural areas where firearms are more accessible (Cantor & Slater 1995).

A number of factors that may be fundamental to suicide behaviour include a propensity to maladaptive coping behaviours, personal vulnerability and the relative lethality of these behaviours. Most distressed individuals do not respond with self-destructive behaviour.

Of those that do respond to life events by engaging in suicidal behaviour, the majority do not die because their behaviour does not generate the necessary lethality. Hence, suicide can be said to be the product of a number of fundamentals—vulnerability, self-destructive responses to a stressor and lethality of those behavioural responses. In a recent research study the authors summarise their findings as follows (Cantor & Baume 1998):

- An increased availability of a culturally accepted method of suicide tends to result in an increase in the suicide rate for that method.
- Restricting the availability of a particular method of suicide tends to result in a corresponding decline in suicide rates for that method.
- Restricting the availability of a particular method of suicide often, but not invariably, reduces overall suicide rates. A complex interaction of factors will determine this outcome. There has been a tendency to neglect the influences of independently evolving methods of suicide.
- Changing the cultural acceptability of the method of suicide will influence suicide rates by that method and may alter overall suicide rates.

Although considerable scope exists for reducing suicides by firearms, motor vehicle exhaust and poisoning by solids and liquids, reduction of suicide by hanging remains very difficult, if not insurmountable. The current tightening of firearm legislation may contribute to the reduction in suicide by this method. However, Cantor, Turrell and Baume (1996) also call for a range of measures that may limit access to lethal medications that are frequently used for suicide. In addition there is scope for reducing motor vehicle suicides. One strategy is to develop tighter standards for catalytic converters, which reduce the carbon monoxide content of exhaust gas. Further methods include the possible introduction of carbon monoxide sensors within cars (which may sound an alarm or switch off the engine if ambient carbon monoxide reaches dangerous levels) and exhaust pipe modifications (making it more difficult to insert a hose into the exhaust pipe) (Routley & Ozanne-Smith 1998; Skopek & Perkins 1998). While it will never be possible to prevent all suicides by such approaches, reasonable cost-effective measures may give suicidal individuals second chances and spare family and friends from considerable grief.

ATTEMPTED SUICIDES

Most information collected about suicide does not include data on suicide attempts. The Australian Bureau of Statistics (1998) reports hospital separations for suicide attempts but there are reliability problems with hospital coding of suicide attempts and most do not present to hospital. Suicidal ideation is even more difficult to study because researchers must rely on self-report from surveys or interviews.

For the reasons noted above a true picture of attempted suicide is not available at this time. Traditionally the rates for females have always been estimated to be several times the rate of males. However, as seen in Figure 5.7, the rates are actually closer. Recently, the male to female ratio of hospital presentations for attempted suicide in Australia has been reported to be approximately 1.4 to 1 (AIHW 1994).

The prevalence of suicide attempts, however, is believed to be grossly under-estimated because most research records only hospital contact. Studies generally have estimated that the ratio between non-lethal suicidal behaviour and suicide varies between 20:1 and 100:1. It is expected that the ratio varies according to age, sex and other factors, such as the operational definition used for suicide attempt which seems to vary from one emergency department to the next.

There is a small sub-set of people who use suicidal behaviour as a habitual pattern of response to stressful events. Repeaters are more likely to die by suicide than those who attempt only once. The prevalence of suicide attempt is much higher than completed suicides, with a statistical probability of up to 60 times for the general population. Studies suggest that 25 to 40% of people who complete suicide have made at least one previous attempt (Kosky 1987).

Figure 5.7 Hospital separation rates due to self-injury, by age group: Australia (excluding NT), 1996–97

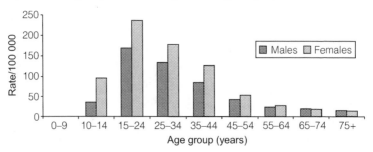

Source: ABS 1998

Rural versus urban suicides

Changes in suicide rates in rural regions, especially for those aged 15 to 24 years, appear even greater than in urban areas. A number of studies have reported significant increases in suicide of young people residing in rural areas, although these increases are not always generalisable to all areas (Baume & Clinton 1997; Baume, Cantor & McTaggart 1998; Dudley et al. 1992; Dudley, Cantor & de Moore 1996). The largest numbers of suicides occurred around the metropolitan areas but the sharpest rate increase occurred in small rural towns. This trend has not been reflected in females except for smaller towns (Dudley et al. 1992). A recent Australian study has found few overall urban/rural differences in suicide rates. This is partly accounted for by small rural regions having both the highest and lowest suicide rates, with low rates found in some relatively affluent rural areas and high rates in more deprived areas (Baume, Cantor & McTaggart 1998).

Although human beings are generally seen to adapt to a great variety of stressors in a relatively short period of time, certain life events may affect or challenge an already vulnerable person (Cassileth et al. 1984; Ormel 1983). One such event, which may account for a more severe rise in the rates for those geographical areas, has been the movement of young people away from small rural towns. A number of authors have asserted that young people moving away to rural cities or to the coastal areas may be protected by a number of factors. Personal characteristics of those moving, or comparatively resource-rich destinations may protect them, whereas those left behind in or migrating to rural inland areas may endure adverse circumstances or may be personally more susceptible to suicide (Baume & Clinton 1997; Dudley, Cantor & de Moore 1996). Suicidal behaviour is often associated with interpersonal factors such as a previous or a recent significant loss (Marttunen et al. 1994) and often reflects family turmoil, turmoil rendered even more tragic when a suicide occurs. This continues a kind of vicious circle of negative events which may lead to other suicides occurring in that family or neighbouring communities as well as increased risks of other problems (Calhoun, Selby & Selby 1982; DeVries, Dalla Lana & Falck 1994; Shneidman 1969).

The above issues bring into question whether the difficulties observed in young suicidal people are purely psychosocial in nature as a reaction to life events, or if a more definite personal vulnerability, where the suicidal person is less resilient and displays a less mature coping style, may be identified. The interpersonal difficulties preceding suicidal behaviour (Andrews & Lewinsohn 1992; Moscicki 1994; Shaffer et al.

1988) may not merely be the result of situational conflicts. They may be part of a personal vulnerability, where the young person living in a rural area is somehow less resilient and less able to cope with certain life events, which influence the way they react to difficult situations. Such a situation may be made more difficult with isolation and lack of access to services, or when the socialisation process focuses on reinforcing a behaviour which negates the value of personal feeling and condones heavy drinking or aggressive behaviour (Baume & Clinton 1997; Baume, Cantor & McTaggart 1998).

Young people in rural communities may also be at risk for a range of mental health problems, stress related illnesses and overuse of prescribed drugs (Bryant 1992; Lawrence 1987) as well as a higher rate of alcohol consumption than their metropolitan counterparts. Higher rates of alcohol abuse are often related, at least in part, to a higher level of domestic violence, sexual assault and incest in certain rural areas (Yellowlees & Kaushik 1994). Substance abuse in young males has been linked to suicidal behaviour (Lipschitz 1995). Young people residing in rural areas also have greater access to firearms and rural communities have proportionally greater levels of suicide by firearms (Baume, Cantor & McTaggart 1998; Cantor & Slater 1995; Cantor, Turrell & Baume 1996; Wallace 1986).

RISK FACTORS

Suicides are the outcomes of self-determined acts. There has been much discussion about the reasons why many people die by suicide. Suicide is the culmination of a series of very complex events. Its origins are multifactorial. An understanding of these factors may therefore assist our appreciation of this complex phenomenon and guide the management of suicidal behaviour with this group of individuals. These include, but are not limited to, socio-cultural factors, individual factors, mental illness, imitations and predisposing family factors. A summary or risk factors is given in Table 5.3.

Socio-cultural factors

Durkheim regarded the state of society as an important element in the genesis of suicide and tended to dismiss the effect of mental illness or stressful life events on the individual. In his view, cohesion reduced suicidal activity within the community, while anomie promoted it (Durkheim 1951). Social and cultural factors usually include the

Table 5.3   Risk factors for suicide

Individual	Social/environmental
• Poor problem solving skills • Low self-esteem • Feelings of hopelessness • Situational crisis • Recent relationship break up • Substance abuse • Sense of failure	• Unemployment • Recent job loss • Changes in lifestyle • Poor access to services • Non-supportive environment • Living alone • Conflict in environment • Legal problems
Predisposing/historical	Mental
• Chronic pain • Child abuse • Exposure to suicide • Previous attempt • Previous suicide in the family • Previous loss	• Depression • Alcoholism • Conduct/personality disorder • Schizophrenia • History of mental illness

Source: Baume, McTaggart & Cantor 1997

general state of social demoralisation or fragmentation, permissive social attitudes towards suicide, media attention to celebrated suicides, social isolation from a supportive network, suicidal role models of peers, unemployment, and/or an environment that facilitates suicide, such as one that permits the ready availability of certain lethal means (Hassan 1995). All of these appear to influence the suicide rates with suicides not limited to a particular socio-economic class. A high level of psychiatric morbidity and lack of access to resources may further increase the risk for those who are socially disadvantaged and facing high levels of life stress such as a recent loss, unemployment or physical illness (Heikkinen et al. 1997; Morrell et al. 1993).

Mental illness and suicide

Existing evidence indicates that although no single determinant is either necessary or sufficient to bring about suicide, mental illness is more common in populations of people completing suicide, with suicide and suicidal behaviours occurring much more frequently in populations of psychiatric patients (Kosky 1998). Retrospective studies based on psychological autopsies and on record linkage have been conducted in various countries. The majority of these studies report the presence of a mental illness or recent history of mental disorder in up to 90% of persons who die by suicide (Harris & Barraclough 1997).

Of the psychiatric disorders, depressive illnesses are the most common. Affective disorders consistently have been found to be associated with suicidal ideation, suicide attempts and completed suicide at a much higher rate than non clinical populations. Recent research has identified depression to be present in 30 to 70% of individuals who completed suicide (Lesage et al. 1994). Other disorders found more commonly among suicide completers than in the general population include substance abuse disorders (especially alcoholism), schizophrenia, personality disorders and, to a lesser extent, anxiety disorders and eating disorders. However, there are large variations among studies addressing the suicide risk in these populations, with estimates ranging from 15 to 75 times the risk found in the general population (Brent et al. 1990).

Imitations

A large number of studies have supported the hypothesis that there is a significant relationship between the reporting of suicide and subsequent suicides. These include those who have examined the link between media reports about suicide and subsequent suicides (Gould & Shaffer 1986; Phillips 1978, 1986; Skopek & Perkins 1998; Wasserman 1984). A number of authors have reported clustering of suicides (Berman 1988; Gould & Davidson 1988; Martin 1992), which suggests that imitation occurs following media coverage or personal contact with the suicide event (Church & Phillips 1984; Goldney 1989; Niemi 1975; Shaffer 1974). Media reports have been demonstrated to significantly influence young people to complete suicide (Hassan 1995). More recently and of greater concern, owing to its immense capacity as well as its lack of formal control, studies have reported the negative impact of the internet on suicide (Baume, Cantor & Rolfe 1997). This evidence supports the view that if suicide is discussed and described explicitly in a public forum, vulnerable young people may consider it a viable option. Hence young people who are struggling with seemingly insurmountable personal, inter-personal or family problems may be the most vulnerable when confronted by the news of the suicide of a celebrity or a close friend (Baume & Clinton 1997; Lester 1992a; Shaffer et al. 1988).

Risk factors and family dynamics

Attempted suicide has been noted more frequently in young people than in older people (see Figure 5.7). Long term follow-up studies have found that 10 to 13% of attempters ultimately take their lives (Tousignant, Bastien & Hamel 1993). Studies have also found

Figure 5.8 Relative risk estimates for suicide in the 14 to 24 year age group: Western Australia, 1968–88

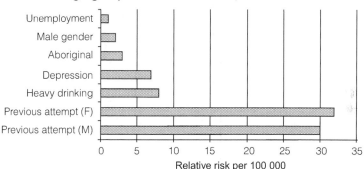

Source: Kosky, Silburn & Zubrick 1990

that suicide attempts are one of the strongest predictors of completed suicide (see Figure 5.8). Evidence, therefore, tends to suggest that suicidal behaviour increases the risk of eventual death by suicide, and is likely to place additional stress on those families. These events may in turn increase their vulnerabilities to life events.

In terms of family background, much evidence suggests that conflict and turmoil are common in environments where previous suicide attempts have taken place. Wenz (1979) characterised the early home environment of the attempted suicide as a family anomie syndrome. Additionally, the lack of secure attachments in childhood has also been highlighted. Sakinofsky (1978) reported that 60% of attempted suicides have a history of chaotic family background, marked by dissension, separations, divorce or parental death and child abuse. Particular familial stressors that have been implicated in the suicide of young persons include, but are not limited to, conflict with parents, loss of significant relationship, child abuse, and loss of a parent, especially due to divorce (Stuart, Klinidis & Minas 1997).

The issue of social adaptability has also been raised as a potential factor affecting an already vulnerable person. Impaired social skills and poor familial relationships are often associated with suicide. Further, a strong relationship has been found between chronically impaired social adjustment, depression, and suicide. A relationship between parental loss and increased risk of suicide has been found in many studies. Kosky (1987) found that 80% of young suicidal people with chronic mental illness had suffered the death of a parent, compared to 20% of a non-suicidal psychiatric control group.

CONCLUSION

The event of a person's death through suicide has significant reper-
cussions for society, as well as for the family of the deceased. It has
been illustrated that the incidence of suicide, particularly in the young
population aged less than 30 years, is rising and that this increase is
reflected worldwide and within metropolitan and rural areas of Australia. Suicide is a complex human behaviour that represents the
confluence of psychological, biological and environmental vulnerabilities. The overlap of multiple contributory risk factors explored in this
chapter influence the expression of suicidal behaviour in particular
individuals and helps explain why a number of people suffering from
specific psychological distress will end their lives by suicide. Suicide
is a behavioural outcome, where the suicidal individual, often feeling
humiliated, suffering from a mental illness that has not been well
managed, and having few social supports, can no longer imagine any
other possibility than to end the pain and despair of living. In this
way, hopelessness appears to be a key mediating factor in suicidal
behaviour. As health professionals, nurses have a role and obligation
to use knowledge and skills to try to avert a person carrying out a
suicidal act.

It is hoped that the information presented here will assist nurses
with new knowledge as well as data derived from Australian sources.
It was not the author's purpose to provide a specific management
template, as this would require a separate and specific chapter. Nursing
of persons with suicidal behaviour is not limited to mental health
nurses. The information provided here should complement government hospital policies already in place or presently being introduced.
Caring for suicidal people and their families should be a holistic
process, based on a spirit of cooperation with other disciplines/services
to improve its effectiveness.

REFERENCES

Andrews, J.A. and Lewinsohn, P.M. (1992) 'Suicidal attempts among older adolescents:
    Prevalence and co-occurence with psychiatric disorders', *Journal of the American
    Academy of Child and Adolescent Psychiatry*, vol. 31, pp. 655–62.
Australian Bureau of Statistics (ABS) (1998) *Cause of Death—Australia, 1997* cat. no.
    3303.0, Canberra: AGPS.
Australian Institute of Health and Welfare (1994) *Australia's Health*, Canberra: AGPS.
Baume, P.J.M. (1988) 'Perspectives on youth suicide', *The Australian Journal of Advanced
    Nursing*, vol. 5, pp. 40–8.

Baume, P.J.M. (1995) 'Youth suicide: Australia's shame', *Hospital and Health Care*, vol. 6, pp. 30–2,

Baume, P.J.M., Cantor, C.H. and McTaggart, P. (1998) *Suicides in Queensland: A Comprehensive Study: 1990–1995*, Brisbane: Australian Academic Press.

Baume, P.J.M., Cantor, C.H. and Rolfe, A. (1997) 'Cybersuicide: The role of interactive suicide notes on the internet', *Crisis*, vol. 18, no. 2, pp. 71–9.

Baume, P.J.M. and Clinton, M. (1997) 'Social and cultural patterns of suicide in young people in rural Australia', *Australian Journal of Rural Health*, vol. 5, no. 3, pp. 115–20.

Baume, P.J.M., McTaggart, P. and Cantor, C.H. (1997) 'Suicide in Australia: Epidemiology and impact', *Suicide Research Bulletin*, vol. 1, no. 1, pp. 1–9.

Baume, P.J.M. and Snowdon, J (1999) 'Managing suicidal behaviour and depression in the elderly', *Australian Suicide Research Bulletin*, Sydney: Adis International.

Beck, A.T., Steer, R.A., Beck, J.S. and Newman, C.F. (1993) 'Hopelessness, depression, suicidal ideation, and clinical diagnosis of depression', *Suicide and Life-Threatening Behaviour*, vol. 23, no. 2, pp. 139–45.

Berman, A. (1988) 'Fictional depiction of suicide in television films and imitation effects', *American Journal of Psychiatry*, vol. 145, no. 8, pp. 982–6.

Brent, D.A., Kolko, D.J., Allan, M.J. and Brown, R.V. (1990) 'Suicidality in affectively disordered adolescent inpatients', *Journal of the American Academy of Child and Adolescent Psychiatry*, vol. 29, pp. 586–93.

Bryant, L. (1992) 'Social aspects of the farm crisis', in Lawrence, G., Vanclay, F. and Furze, B. (eds) *Agriculture, Environment and Society: Contemporary Issues for Australia*, Melbourne: Macmillan, pp. 157–72.

Buckley, N.A., Whyte, I.M., Dawson, A.H., McManus, P.R. and Ferguson, P.R. (1995a) 'Self-poisoning in Newcastle, 1987–1992', *Medical Journal of Australia*, vol. 162, pp. 190–3.

Buckley, N.A., Whyte, I.M., Dawson, A.H., McManus, P.R. and Ferguson, P.R. (1995b) 'Correlations between prescriptions and drugs taken in self-poisoning: Implications for prescribers and drug regulation', *Medical Journal of Australia*, vol. 162, pp. 194–7.

Burvill, P. W. (1998) 'Migrant suicide rates in Australia and in country of birth', *Psychological Medicine*, vol. 28, no. 1, pp. 201–8.

Calhoun, L.G., Selby, J.W. and Selby, L.E. (1982) 'The psychological aftermath of suicide: An analysis of current evidence', *Clinical Psychology Review*, vol. 2, pp. 409–20.

Cantor, C.H. and Baume, P.J.M. (1998) 'Access to methods of suicide: What impact?', *Australian and New Zealand Journal of Psychiatry*, vol. 32, pp. 8–14.

Cantor, C.H. and Slater, P.J. (1995) 'The impact of firearm control legislation on suicide in Queensland: Preliminary findings', *The Medical Journal of Australia*, vol. 162, pp. 583–5.

Cantor, C.H., Turrell, G. and Baume, P.J.M. (1996) *Access to Means of Suicide by Young Australians*, A background report prepared for the Commonwealth Department of Health and Family Services, Youth Suicide Prevention Advisory Group, Canberra.

Cassileth, B.R., Lusk, E.J., Strouse, T.B., Miller, D.S., Brown, L.L., Cross, P.A. and Tenaglia, A.N. (1984) 'Psychological status in chronic illness: A comparative analysis of six diagnostic groups', *New England Journal of Medicine*, no. 311, pp. 506–11.

Church, I. and Phillips, J. (1984) 'Suggestion and suicide by plastic bag asphyxia', *British Journal of Psychiatry*, vol. 144, pp. 100–1.

DeVries, B., Dalla Lana, R. and Falck, V.T. (1994) 'Parental bereavement over the life course: A theoretical intersection and empirical review', *Omega*, vol. 29, no. 1, pp. 47–69.

Diekstra, R. and Garnefski, M. (1995) 'On the nature, the gravity and causality of suicide', *Suicide and Life-Threatening Behaviour*, vol. 25, no. 1, pp. 36–57.

Dudley, M., Cantor, C. and de Moore, G. (1996) 'Jumping the gun: Firearms and the mental health of Australians', *Australian and New Zealand Journal of Psychiatry*, vol. 30, pp. 370–81.

Dudley, M.J., Keld, N.J, Florida, T.M., Harvard, J.P. and Waters, B.G. (1998) 'Suicide among young Australians, 1964–1993: An interstate comparison of urban and rural trends', *Medical Journal of Australia*, no. 169, pp. 77–80.

Dudley, M., Waters, B., Kelk, N. and Howard, J. (1992) 'Youth suicide in New South Wales: Urban rural trends', *Medical Journal of Australia*, vol. 156, pp. 83–8.

Durkheim, E., (1951) *Suicide: A Study in Sociology*, Glencoe: Free Press (original work published 1897).

Farmer, K.A. (1996) 'Medically serious suicide attempts in jails with a suicide prevention programme', *Journal of Forensic Science*, vol. 41, no. 2, pp. 240–6.

Fedden, H.R. (1980) *Suicide: A Social and Historical Study*, New York: Arno Press.

Freud, S. (1964) *Mourning and Melancholia*; Collected Papers, vol. 4, London: Hogarth Press.

Goldney R. (1989) 'Suicide: The role of the media', *Australian and New Zealand Journal of Psychiatry*, vol. 23, pp. 30–4.

Gould, M. and Davidson, L. (1988) 'Suicide contagion among adolescents', in Stillman, A. & Feldman, R. (eds) *Advances in Mental Health, Volume III: Depression and Suicide*, Greenwich: JAI Press.

Gould, M. and Shaffer, D. (1986) 'The impact of suicide in television movies', *New England Journal of Medicine*, vol. 315, pp. 690–4.

Hallenstein, A. (1994) 'The prevention of suicide', Draft Report No. 1, Canberra: NH&MRC.

Harris, E.C. and Barraclough, B. (1997) 'Suicide as an outcome for mental disorders: A meta-analysis', *The British Journal of Psychiatry*, vol. 170, pp. 205–28.

Hassan, R. (1995) *Suicide Explained: The Australian Experience*, Melbourne: Melbourne University Press.

Heikkinen, M.E., Henriksson, M.M., Isometsa, E.T., Marttunen, M.J., Aro, H.M. and Lonquist, J.K. (1997) 'Recent life events and suicide personality disorders', *Journal of Nervous and Mental Disorders*, vol. 195, no. 6, pp. 373–81.

Hunter, E. (1993) *Aboriginal Health and History: Power and Privilege in Remote Australia*, Melbourne: Cambridge University Press.

Jones, A.L., Hayes, P.C., Proudfoot, A.T., Vale, J.A., Prescott, L.F. and Krauzelok, E.P. (1997) 'Should methionine be added to every paracetamol tablet?', *British Medical Journal*, vol. 315, no. 7103, pp. 301–4.

Kosky, R. (1987) 'Is suicide behaviour increasing among Australian youth', *Medical Journal of Australia*, 17 August, vol. 147, no. 4, pp. 164–6.

Kosky, R. (1998) 'Suicide: Rational or irrational?', *Australian Psychiatry*, vol. 6, pp. 17–19.

Kosky, R., Silburn, S. & Subrick, S. (1990) 'Are children and adolescents who have suicidal thoughts different from those who attempt suicide?', *Journal of Nervous and Mental Disorders*, January, vol. 128, no. 1, pp. 38–43.

Lawrence, G. (1987) *Capitalism and the Countryside: The Rural Crisis in Australia*, Sydney: Pluto.

Lesage, A.D., Boyer, R., Grunberg, F., Vanier, C., Morissette, R., Menard-Buteau, C. and Loywer, M. (1994) 'Suicide and mental disorders: A case control study of young men', *American Journal of Psychiatry*, vol. 151, no. 7, pp. 1063–8.

Lester, D. (1992a). *Why People Kill Themselves: A 1990s Summary of Research Findings on Suicidal Behavior*, Springfield, IL: Charles C. Thomas.

Lester, D. (1992b) 'Alcoholism and drug abuse' in Maris, R.W., Berman, A.L., Maltsberger, J.T. and Yufit, R.I. (eds) *Assessment and Prediction of Suicide* New York: Guildford Press, pp. 32–36.

Lipschitz, A. (1995) 'Suicide prevention in young adults', *Suicide & Life-Threatening Behaviour*, vol. 25, p. 1.

Martin, G. (1992) 'Adolescent suicide 3: Imitation and clustering phenomenon', *Youth Studies Australia*, vol. 11, no. 1, pp. 28–32.

Marttunen, M., Avro, H., Henriksson, M. and Lonquist, J. (1994) 'Antisocial behaviour in adolescent suicide', *Acta Psychiatrica Scandinavica*, vol. 89, pp. 167–73.

McDonald, B. and Steel, Z. (1997) *Immigrants and Mental health: An Epidemiological Analysis*, Sydney: Transcultural Mental Health Centre.

Mina, E.S. and Gallop, R. (1998) 'Chilhood sexual and physical abuse and adult self-harm and suicidal behaviour', *Canadian Journal of Psychiatry*, vol. 43, pp. 793–800.

Morrell, S., Taylor, R., Quine, S. and Kerr, C. (1993) 'Suicide and unemployment in Australia 1901–1990', Journal of Social Science and Medicine, vol. 36, no. 6, pp. 749–6.

Moscicki, E.K. (1994) 'Gender differences in completed and attempted suicides', *Annals of Epidemiology*, vol. 4, no. 2, pp. 152–8.

Niemi, T. (1975) 'The time-space distances of suicides committed in the lock-up in Finland in 1963–67', *Psychiatria Fennica*, pp. 267–70.

Ormel, J. (1983) 'Neuroticism and well-being inventories: Measuring traits or states?', *Psychological Medicine*, vol. 13, pp. 165–76.

Phillips, D. (1978). 'Motor vehicle fatalities increase just after publicised suicide stories', *Science*, vol. 196, pp. 1464–6.

Phillips, D. (1986). 'Natural experiments on the effects of mass media violence on fatal aggression', *Advances in Experimental Social Psychology*, vol. 19, pp. 139–45.

Phillips, D.P. and Bollen, K.A. (1985) 'Same time last year: Selective data dredging for negative findings', *American Sociological Review*, vol. 50, pp. 364–71.

Phillips, D.P. and Carstensen, L.L. (1986) 'Clustering of teenage suicides after television news stories about suicide', *New England Journal of Medicine*, vol. 315, no. 11, pp. 685–9.

Phillips, D.P., Lesyna, K. and Paight, D.J. (1992) 'Suicide and the media', in Maris, R.W., Berman, A.L., Maltsberger, J.T. and Yufit, R.I. (eds) *Assessment and Prediction of Suicide*, New York: Guildford Press, pp. 499–519.

Phillips, D.P. and Paight, D.J. (1987) 'The impact of televised movies about suicide', *New England Journal of Medicine*, vol. 317, pp. 809–11.

Pritchard, C. (1992) 'Youth suicide and gender in Australia and New Zealand compared with countries of the Western World 1973–1987', *Australian and New Zealand Journal of Psychiatry*, vol. 26, pp. 609–17.

Routley, V. and Ozanne-Smith, J. (1998) 'The impact of catalytic converters on motor vehicle exhaust gas suicides', *The Medical Journal of Australia*, vol. 168, no. 2, pp. 65–8.

Sakinofsky, I. (1978) 'Life situations and lifestyles of persons who attempt suicide', Paper presented at the 11th Annual Meeting of the American Association of Suicidology, New Orleans, LA.

Shaffer D. (1974) 'Suicide in childhood and early adolescence', *Journal of Child Psychology and Psychiatry*, vol. 15, pp. 275–91.

Shaffer, D., Garland, A., Gould, M., Fisher, P. and Trautman, P. (1988) 'Preventing teenage suicide: A critical review', *Journal of American Academy of Child Adolescence Psychiatry*, vol. 27, no. 6, pp. 675–87.

Shneidman, E. (1969) *On the Nature of Suicide*, San Francisco: Jossey-Bass.

Shneidman, E. (1993) *Suicide as a Psychache*, Hillsdale, NU: Aronson.

Skopek, M.A. and Perkins, R. (1998) 'Deliberate exposure to motor vehicle exhaust gas: The psychosocial profile of attempted suicide', *Australian and New Zealand Journal of Psychiatry*, vol. 32, pp. 830–8.

Stuart, G.W., Klinidis, S. and Minas, I.H. (1997) 'The treated prevalence of mental disorder amongst immigrants and the Australian-born: Community and primary care rates', *International Journal of Social Psychiatry*, vol. 44, no. 1, pp. 22–34.

Tousignant, M., Bastien, M.F. and Hamel, S. (1993) 'Suicidal attempts and ideations among adolescents and young adults: The role of father's and mother's care of parental separation', *Social Psychiatry and Psychiatric Epidemiology*, vol. 28, no. 5, pp. 256–61.

UNICEF (1996) *The Progress of Nations, 1996*, New York: UNICEF.

Wallace, A. (1986) *Homicide: The Social Reality*, Sydney: New South Wales Bureau of Crime Statistics & Research.

Wasserman, I. (1984) 'Imitation and suicide: A re-examination of the effect', *American Sociology Review*, vol. 49, pp. 427–36.

Wenz, F.V. (1979) 'Self-injury behavior, economic status and the family anomie syndrome among adolescents', *Adolescence*, vol. 14, no. 54, pp. 387–98.

Yellowlees, P. and Kaushik, A. (1994) 'An examination of the association between life problems and psychiatric disorders in a rural patient population', *Australian and New Zealand Journal of Psychiatry*, vol. 28, pp. 50–7.

COMMENTARY—CHAPTER 5

Jennifer Chipps & Beverley Raphael

Suicide is a complex and tragic phenomenon. Although this chapter provides an interesting and broad overview of suicide, there is a need to provide better guidance to the roles of nurses in suicide prevention and how suicide data can inform and assist nurses in everyday practice.

Health services act as contact areas for people at risk of suicide: suicide deaths, though tragic, are relatively rare. The biggest problems that face nurses are individuals who present with a range of suicidal behaviours, including behaviour in which the intent to die is not obvious. It is estimated that for every suicide death recorded that 30 to 40 people may attempt suicide[1] and as many as 90 to 120 people may think of suicide.[2] Individuals with possible suicidal behaviours, specifically previous suicide attempts, are at increased risk of subsequent death by suicide. While not all suicides can be prevented, appropriate intervention at the right time may prevent many of them.

Individuals at risk of possible suicidal behaviour present in a range of health settings such as emergency departments, general wards, the community, mental health inpatient units and general health services such as youth health services and postnatal services.[3] Nurses, both in the general and in the mental health disciplines, are the main groups of health professionals in these settings. When assistance is sought for suicidal behaviour, including suicidal threats, the nurse's response must be prompt, effective, and based on local policies and procedures that reflect evidence-based and culturally appropriate practice. Competent management when the individual presents with possible suicidal behaviour will have a significant influence on both morbidity and mortality outcomes.

The assessment and management of suicide is a mental health responsibility. Up to 90% of people who die from suicide have a diagnosable mental health problem at the time of their death and depression is one of the most common.[4] Depression (as with most mental health problems) is treatable and preventable. It is therefore essential that every person who presents to health services with possible suicidal behaviour has a suicide risk assessment followed by a mental health assessment. Assessment for depression, a common condition, should become routine in most health settings. Nurses can play a vital role in these assessment and management processes, more so as they are likely to be the frontline health professionals dealing with individuals at risk of suicide.

Mental health clients in Australia have much the same suicide risk (ten times that of the general population) as mental health clients in systems of care overseas.[5] However, transition periods in care are periods of increased suicide risk with individuals recently discharged from mental health units being 100 to 200 times more at risk of suicide than the general population.[6] This increased risk relates to changes in support, changes in levels of supervision, non-adherence to treatment regimes and possible return to stressful environments. Appropriate assertive follow up of these patients is essential. Nurses, in both their engagement in care provision and in their commitment to quality and continuity of care, can provide a strong focus for better outcomes for these clients.

Increasingly nurses also play active roles in planning and delivering suicide prevention programs. Developing these programs involves identifying effective means to address the range of risk and protective factors associated with suicide. Not all suicide prevention initiatives will directly address suicide, but many will address some of the risk factors: mental health problems such as depression and other stressors such as failing at school, unemployment, relationship break up and family conflict. Other initiatives will address protective factors such as personal resilience and supportive relationships. These initiatives may also target younger children many years before they are likely to attempt suicide and when suicide risk factors begin to develop. Nurses can play an active role in these programs within schools or within the community.

ENDNOTES

1   NH&MRC (1993) *Scope for Prevention in Mental Health*, Commonwealth of Australia.

2   Sayer, G., Stewart, G. and Chipps, J. (1996) 'Suicide attempts in NSW: Associated mortality and morbidity', *NSW Public Health Bulletin*, vol. 7, no. 6, pp. 55–63.

3   Circular 98/31: Policy guidelines for the management of patients with possible suicidal behaviour for NSW Health Staff and staff of private health facilities, NSW Department of Health, 1998.

4   Henriksson, M.M., Aro, H.M., Heikinen, M.E., Isometsa, E.T., Kuoppasalmi, K.I. and Lonnqvist, J.K. (1993) 'Mental disorders and comorbidity in suicide', *American Journal of Psychiatry*, vol. 150, no. 6, pp. 935–40.

5   Chipps, J., Stewart, G. and Sayer, G. (1995) 'Suicide mortality in NSW: Clients of mental health services', *NSW Public Health Bulletin*, vol. 6, no. 8, pp. 75–81.

6   Gunnell, D. and Frankel, S. (1994) 'Prevention of suicide: Aspirations and evidence', *British Medical Journal*, vol. 308, pp. 1227–30; Chipps, J., Stewart, G. and Sayer, G. (1995) 'Suicide mortality in New South Wales: Clients of mental health services', *NSW Public Health Bulletin*, vol. 6, no. 8, pp. 75–81.

6   Drug use

Kate Dolan

INTRODUCTION

Why some drugs are legal and others are not has more to do with history than with the drugs themselves (Manderson 1993). Drug use and opposition to it are not recent events. People have been taking drugs for thousands of years. Opium use is thought to have originated in Mesopotamia over 7000 years ago and hallucinogenic mushrooms were used by the Hindu in ancient times. However, the use of these substances was generally restricted to ceremonies. According to Lang (1998), there are no accounts of widespread recreational use of drugs other than alcohol and tobacco before the opium epidemic in the eighteenth and nineteenth centuries. Lang suggests that such drug use did occur but went unrecorded as it did not pose a threat to the existing social order (1998, p. 2). Anti-drug campaigns are known to have occurred since the sixteenth century. To aim for a drug free society is somewhat naive. Rather, the challenge is to accept that some level of drug use is inevitable and to minimise the harm resulting from use.

TYPES OF DRUGS AND THEIR EFFECTS

There are three basic types of drugs—stimulants, depressants and hallucinogens; as their names suggest, they produce stimulating, depressing or hallucinogenic effects (Jacobs & Fehr 1987).

Stimulants

Amphetamines were developed in the 1920s in the United States. In the 1960s, amphetamines were used to treat depression and obesity and are still prescribed today, but only for a few conditions such as attention deficit disorder in children. Amphetamines come in a powder form and are usually inhaled through the nose (snorted) or injected.

Amphetamines increase central nervous system activity. Acute amphetamine poisoning (overdose) can cause a number of effects including irregular heart beat, heart attack, a very high fever and burst blood vessels in the brain. At high doses, amphetamines can create a toxic psychosis characterised by paranoid delusions, hallucinations and aggressive behaviour. Long term injection of amphetamines can result in a blockage of blood vessels (caused by the contaminants mixed in them), which can lead to major damage to the body's organs and inflamed blood vessels and abscesses. Regular use can produce chronic sleeping problems, anxiety, appetite suppression, high blood pressure and skin rashes. There is a feeling of confidence, but it can be unpredictable and cause agitation or even violent behaviour.

Cocaine, one well-known amphetamine, is derived from the coca plant and was available from chemists until the early 1920s as a local anaesthetic for minor surgery and as a 'pick me up', or tonic. Cocaine also comes in a powder form and is snorted or injected. Initially the effects of cocaine are euphoric, with users becoming talkative and active. Excessive amounts, however, can cause headaches and dizziness as well as heart failure, respiratory problems and overdose. The 'high' from the drug is very brief and repeated doses are needed to maintain the high. Cocaine injectors can inject up to ten or 15 times a day. In the short term, low doses of cocaine may induce tremor and muscle twitches and, in severe cases, even seizures. After the euphoric effects have faded, the user is left in a severe state of agitation. There is anxiety, rapid flight of ideas, feelings of grandiosity and paranoid ideation. With regular use the user may suffer from paranoid psychosis. In the long term, the user will appear nervous and agitated. There can be hypersensitivity to sensory stimuli, to the point of hallucination. A common hallucination is of insects crawling under the skin, which leads to frantic scratching to the point where the skin is broken and infection is common.

Depressants

Heroin is a narcotic analgesic, meaning that it is a very strong pain-killer. Heroin is manufactured from morphine, which is derived from opium. In the early 1900s, heroin was legally sold as a cure for coughs. It stimulates the brain resulting in a depression of activity in the central nervous system, subsequently affecting balance, concentration and coordination. Heroin, when used hygienically and in pure form, is not especially toxic and appears to cause little damage to the user's body. However, as heroin is usually used by injection it can be harmful, especially if the procedure is not sterile. Initial reactions to heroin include vomiting and nausea. Immediately after an injection of heroin, the user feels a surge of pleasure or 'rush' that gives way to a state of gratification. Other immediate effects include relief of pain, euphoria, a suppression of coughing, depression of bowel activity and a lower rate of breathing. Users may enter a mild dozing state often referred to as 'the nod'. One side effect of heroin use is lowered sex drive and even impotence in men; in women, it can cause irregular menstruation and sometimes infertility. The combination of injecting heroin and consuming other central nervous system depressants (such as alcohol or tranquillisers) presents a high risk of overdose that can be fatal. Generally the desired effects are only fully appreciated after users acquire tolerance. However, acquisition of tolerance then requires the use of more drugs to achieve the same effects.

Injecting a drug, regardless of the type of drug, presents particular problems. For example there is the risk of acquiring a blood borne viral infection such as HIV, hepatitis B or hepatitis C when injecting equipment is shared among users. There are also other complications from injecting such as abscesses, thrombophlebitis, endocarditis and septicaemia.

Hallucinogens

The leaves, flowering tops and resin of the cannabis plant have been consumed for centuries for their intoxicating effects. The leaves of the cannabis plant are called marijuana. The most common method of consuming cannabis is to roll marijuana into cigarettes called 'joints'. Initial effects of cannabis use include a sense of well-being and relaxation, euphoria, sharpened sensations of taste, smell, touch and hearing. The user's sense of time is distorted. Regular smokers of cannabis may experience sleep disturbances, irritability, restlessness or depression. Concentration, memory and learning abilities may be affected and there may be a decline in motivational levels. Cannabis users may experience an interference in sexual and hormone production. Regular smokers experience a drop in sex drive; men may suffer from a lowered sperm count and women can experience irregular menstrual cycles. On the psychological front there can be psychotic episodes, especially in people who are already predisposed to these conditions. THC, the active ingredient in cannabis, has been shown to be an effective anti-nausea agent for some patients undergoing chemotherapy.

LSD or lysergic acid diethylamide was discovered in 1943 and is manufactured as small tablets or absorbed onto squares of blotting paper which are swallowed. The drug is very potent and only very minute doses are normally taken. It can produce significant changes in perception, mood and thought. Boundaries between self and the environment become blurred. An average 'trip' lasts about 12 hours and may be unpleasant (a bad trip) depending on the surroundings and company. Users can experience flashbacks where they relive the LSD state without having taken more; stress and cannabis use can induce flashbacks. LSD has been used in psychotherapy and in the treatment of alcoholism.

THE NATIONAL DRUG STRATEGY AND DRUG-RELATED RESEARCH

Australia's approach to drugs (illicit and licit) is outlined in the National Drug Strategy, which commenced in 1985. The Strategy has two components—supply reduction measures and demand reduction initiatives—with an overall aim of minimising the harmful effects of drugs on Australian society (Blewett 1987). An independent evaluation of the Strategy in 1997 (Single & Rohl 1997) found that it is one of the most progressive and respected drug strategies in the world. The Strategy includes promotion of partnerships between law enforcement and health departments.

There have been five National Household Surveys of Australians' drug and alcohol use. Between 1985 and 1995, over 15 000 Australians were interviewed, allowing comparisons to be made (Makkai & McAllister 1998)—see Table 6.1. By far the most commonly used drug is alcohol. However, the life-time prevalence of tobacco smoking has declined consistently over the ten year period: about 70% of males and 60% of females report they have smoked tobacco at some time, but only about half this figure are currently smokers.

According to the 1995 National Household Survey, almost 40% of the population aged 14 or more has tried illicit drugs and about half of these did so in the 12 months prior to the survey. Marijuana is the most common illicit drug used in Australia, with one-third of

Table 6.1   National Household Survey, 1995

Drug	% ever used
Alcohol	87
Tobacco	32
Cannabis	31
Heroin	2
Amphetamines	6
Cocaine	3
Hallucinogens	6
Designer drugs—ecstasy	2
Tranquillisers	3*

Note: *non-medical use
Source: Australian Institute of Health and Welfare 1999

respondents having tried it. There were no major changes in the level of drug use since the previous survey in 1993, even though reports of respondents being offered drugs had halved. About 2% of the sample surveyed reported having used heroin at some stage, which is equal to about 170 000 people, within a range of 95 000 to 225 000. However, the survey also found that males are twice as likely to use illicit drugs as females (Makkai & McAllister 1998).

Almost half of the respondents to the 1995 National Household Survey thought that the personal use of marijuana should be legal while less than 10% thought heroin, cocaine or amphetamines should be legal. The use of marijuana was decriminalised in South Australia in 1987 and the Australian Capital Territory in 1992, but its use was no greater than elsewhere in Australia. Marijuana was recently decriminalised in the Northern Territory.

A large scale study, the Inmate Health Survey carried out in 1996, found high levels of drug and alcohol use among prisoners (Butler 1997)— see Table 6.2. Approximately half of the 800 prisoners interviewed reported drinking alcohol at 'harmful' levels prior to entering prison and almost one-third reported having used heroin in the previous year.

Table 6.2   Prisoners' use of alcohol and drugs in the year prior to prison

Drug	% used
Alcohol (at harmful levels)	99 (55)
Cannabis	57
Heroin	32
Amphetamines	27
Cocaine	18

Source: Butler 1997

Illicit drugs and Australian society

Ninety-five per cent of illicit drug deaths are opiate related. There has been an eight fold increase in the rate of opioid overdose mortality from 70 in 1979 to over 600 in 1996 (see Table 6.3). The average age of heroin users dying from drug overdose was 24 in 1979 and 31 in 1995. Possible reasons for the increase in the number of Australians dying from opioid overdoses include an increase in the number of people using heroin; an increase in the purity of heroin; or users are using other drugs such as methadone or benzodiazepines at the same time as they are using heroin.

One of the added dangers of using illicit drugs is the unknown purity and the nature of any adulterants contained in the illicit drugs. While bottles of wine list the alcohol content in standard drinks and cigarette packs list the nicotine content in milligrams, there are no such standards for illicit drugs. Adulterants include a range of substances from talcum powder to refined sugars that can cause damage to the user. The average level of purity in amphetamines in seized street samples is less than 10% and, on average, contaminants comprise 90% of the seized samples. Heroin is sometimes mixed with lactose and quinine.

Pregnant women who use stimulants have a higher rate of miscarriage, premature labour, other complications and underweight babies. Most drugs have some effect on the foetus. There is some evidence that babies of mothers who have used amphetamines and heroin will experience withdrawal symptoms.

Costs of drug use

The mortality and morbidity associated with dependence on opioids have important economic implications for both direct health costs (health care expenditure incurred in treating opiate dependence) and indirect costs (costs incurred by a reduction in the country's economic output resulting from opiate use such as unemployment, crime and absenteeism). It has been estimated that the tangible cost in 1988 of illicit drug use was $1042.4 million and the intangible cost was $398.8 million, making a total of $1441.1 million (Collins & Lapsley 1996). The proportion of the cost of drug abuse attributed to illicit drug use in this particular report is 9%, whereas it is 67% for tobacco and 24% for alcohol.

Table 6.3   Heroin overdoses in Australian jurisdictions, 1994 to 1996

Jurisdiction	1994	1995	1996
NSW	209	273	260
Victoria	97	140	145
Queensland	37	42	32
Western Australia	38	70	64
South Australia	32	38	32
Tasmania	4	6	5
ACT	3	13	17
Northern Territory	5	0	2
Total	**425**	**582**	**557**

Source: Lynskey & Hall 1998

DEPENDENCE ON DRUGS AND WITHDRAWAL

Dependence on drugs can be psychological or physical. The former is characterised by a strong desire to take the drug, an inability to control use, persistent use despite harmful consequences and the prioritisation of drug use over other activities. Physical dependence is characterised by increased tolerance and a physical withdrawal when drug use is discontinued. The frequent use of high doses of drugs may produce tolerance, that is, a state where a higher dose of a drug needs to be taken to achieve the same effects as before.

For example, frequent and heavy users of cannabis may experience a variety of health, social, legal, financial and relationship problems. They may become physically and psychologically dependent on cannabis. Cannabis users may acquire a persistent craving for its psychoactive effects and the drug can become central to their lives. Abrupt termination of use can lead to a mild withdrawal syndrome, including sleep disturbances, irritability, loss of appetite, nervousness, chills, raised temperature, anxiety, sweating and upset stomach. Overall, the symptoms can be described as 'flu' like. The withdrawal sickness usually lasts for less than one week, although the sleep disturbances can last longer.

On the other hand, people can develop tolerance to amphetamines, needing higher doses to achieve the same effects over time. The drug can become central to their thoughts, emotions and activities. Some people use drugs compulsively and find it difficult to stop using or to reduce the amount they are using. Regular use of cocaine can result in dependence and cocaine psychosis. Users may hear voices and feel a sense of persecution. When chronic use is discontinued, the person may feel fatigued, wanting to sleep but experiencing disturbed sleep; however, the appetite is restored. In the first few days of withdrawal a cocaine user may experience these symptoms: exhaustion, increased sleep, depression, restlessness and irritability. Cravings (strong urges to resume drug use) may start, as well as mood swings, disturbed sleep, poor concentration, aches, increased appetite and paranoia.

It takes some time with regular heroin use (weeks and even months) to become dependent on heroin. Increasingly higher doses are needed to produce the desired effects. Users may attempt to reduce the cost of their habit by detoxing, as this reduces their tolerance—less of the drug is needed for the same effect. The severity of withdrawal depends on the extent of the drug use. Opiate withdrawal is uncomfortable, but not life threatening. Common symptoms include: 'goosebumps', profuse sweating, dilated pupils, runny nose, excessive yawning, vomiting, diarrhoea, anorexia, aches and pains, elevated pulse rate and shivering. The onset of symptoms appears eight to 12 hours after the last use of opiates and symptoms reach a peak at 48 to 72 hours.

Detoxification

Detoxification is the process whereby the drug is eliminated from the user's system. It is generally thought of as a prelude to treatment rather than a form of treatment itself. Types of detoxification include medical and non medical. The former is more expensive as medically trained staff are involved while the second is less so as non-medical staff are employed. The main drugs used to deal with opiate withdrawal symptoms include methadone, clonidine and benzodiazepines. A common strategy to assist withdrawal from heroin is provision of decreasing doses of oral methadone. There are now home detoxification programs, where staff visit people at their homes daily to ensure they are medicated sufficiently while they are detoxifying from the drug.

DRUG TREATMENT AND PREVENTION STRATEGIES

This section examines and identifies the current world trends relating to drug treatment and prevention and associated issues.

Primary interventions aim to deter individuals from using illicit drugs, drug education being the most common type of intervention. Syringe exchange can be classified as a primary intervention even though it is targeting current users. The aim of syringe exchange is to prevent infectious diseases rather than to prevent people from injecting.

Secondary interventions target those already using illicit drugs. Examples include motivational interviewing to encourage injecting drug users to think about stopping their drug use and methadone maintenance treatment. For those who continue to use cannabis there are various ways to minimise the harms from using the drug. The risk of respiratory harm can be eliminated by switching from smoking cannabis to either eating it in 'dope cookies' or making tea with it. Those who continue to smoke cannabis can lessen the risk by avoiding deep inhalation and breath holding, both of which are common practices among 'pot' smokers. To minimise the risk of dependence, users can reduce the frequency of use to weekly or even less often. Daily or near daily use has a high risk of producing dependence.

Tertiary interventions aim to rehabilitate those who have suffered from their use of illicit drugs. For injecting drug users, most of the interventions are aimed at opiate users. Some tertiary interventions include: using organisations such as 'narcotics anonymous', methadone maintenance and counselling.

Supply and demand reduction

Supply reduction initiatives typically involve law enforcement agencies to curb the manufacture, importation and distribution of illicit drugs. Demand reduction measures are developed in order to reduce the desire, demand, or need for substances. These demand reduction efforts (such as 'just say no') tend to feature predominately in the public eye, even though they enjoy little success. Early efforts tried to instil fear in potential users of drugs. Approaches now tend to provide balanced information about drugs and their effects. Debate has tended to focus on the relative merits of the supply reduction and demand reduction. One report found that every dollar spent on drug treatment is worth $7 spent on law enforcement (Rydell & Everingham 1994), leading to the conclusion that it is more effective to treat drug users than to arrest and imprison them.

A range of health professionals will come into contact with people who use illicit drugs. Whether or not these people disclose their drug use will depend to an extent on how the professionals present themselves. People with drug problems are more likely to trust health workers who are non judgemental and genuinely helpful. It is important to remember that the use of illicit drugs is an offence and these people may be reluctant to disclose their drug use. Drug using women with children may be especially afraid as they may fear that their children will be removed from them. Some active encouragement is necessary to develop a rapport with people who use illicit drugs. It is also important not to be presumptuous—not all users of illicit drugs have problems.

Harm reduction strategies

Harm reduction strategies in relation to illicit drugs were developed in response to the spread of HIV among injecting drug users in the mid 1980s. Early epidemics of HIV infection among injecting drug users in Edinburgh and New York caused much concern because not only were the people in these groups acquiring HIV but also non injecting drug users who had sexual contact with them. These strategies attempt to reduce the adverse consequences of drug use without necessarily requiring a reduction in consumption of drugs. The user's decision to use drugs is accepted as fact, which does not necessarily mean that it is a decision warranting approval. The user is treated with dignity as a normal person, even though their behaviour may be outside the law. Harm reduction does not necessarily conflict with the goal of abstinence; harm reduction programs can be the first step towards drug treatment. If a person is not willing to give up their drug use, they should be assisted in reducing harm to themselves or others.

Methadone maintenance treatment

Methadone maintenance treatment was introduced in the United States in the 1960s. It has been subjected to hundreds of studies over the years. Methadone maintenance treatment is a substitution therapy for opiate dependent users. Generally clients receive a daily dose which does not produce intoxication once they are stabilised. Methadone clients have superior outcomes in a range of areas, such as avoiding criminal behaviour and mortality, than their untreated peers. It is considered a controversial treatment, because methadone maintenance 'merely' switches dependence to a legal narcotic and also some clients under treatment continue to use heroin and other drugs (Gerstein & Harwood 1990). Methadone clients become much more amenable to counselling and support services that enable them to move away from seeking out and using illicit drugs. (The entire world literature on methadone treatment was recently summarised by Ward, Mattick and Hall in their 1998 book.)

Methadone maintenance treatment is effective in reducing mortality (Caplehorn & Ross 1995), heroin consumption (Gottheil, Sterling

& Weinstein 1993), criminality (Newman & Whitehall 1979) and HIV transmission (Metzger et al. 1993). Methadone maintenance treatment attracts and retains more heroin injectors than any other form of treatment (Ward, Mattick & Hall 1998). Provision of methadone maintenance treatment has rapidly expanded in a number of countries in response to the HIV epidemic. The effectiveness of methadone treatment is dependent on a number of factors including dose (Hubbard et al. 1989) and duration of treatment (Ball & Ross 1991). An increase in methadone places from 19 900 to 34 000 corres-ponded with 24 900 fewer drug arrests and 1500 fewer cases of serum hepatitis in New York City in the early 1970s (Joseph 1988). When methadone maintenance was introduced in Hong Kong in 1976, the annual number of addicts admitted to prison decreased from approximately 2200 to 200 in four years (Joseph 1988).

A study published in 1996 reported that, at that time, there were only seven prison based methadone programs in the world (Dolan & Wodak 1996). A study of the NSW prison methadone program found that when prisoners were provided with adequate methadone treat-ment, self reported heroin injecting and sharing of syringes were significantly lower than for untreated respondents (Dolan, Wodak & Hall 1998). Methadone maintenance treatment in prison can reduce risk behaviours and, therefore, probably also reduce the spread of blood borne infections. The NSW prison methadone program was being studied in 1999 by the National Drug and Alcohol Research Centre.

Needle and syringe programs

A needle and syringe exchange program is a preventive public health treatment which allows the exchange of used needles and syringes for clean ones. Drug users started the first needle and syringe exchange program in the Netherlands in 1984 in response to an increase in hepatitis B infection. Since then, a number of countries have successfully introduced needle and syringe exchange programs (Lurie et al. 1993). One of the most convincing bodies of evidence of the effectiveness of needle and syringe exchange programs comes from a study in the United States. Researchers studied a needle and syringe exchange program for over 18 months. The dates on which almost 2000 needles and syringes were distributed and returned were recorded. Returned syringes were tested for HIV infection. Over time, by mathematical modelling, HIV incidence cases were estimated to have reduced by 33% (Kaplan & O'Keefe 1993). This reduction in HIV incidence did not require reduc-tions in risk behaviour or increases in the number of syringes in circulation. Despite this evidence, needle and syringe exchange programs have only been introduced in a few cities in the United States. However, it has been conservatively estimated that up to 10 000 HIV infections could have been avoided at a cost of US$500 million if syringe exchange had been introduced to United States' cities at the same time and pace as had occurred in Australia (Lurie & Drucker 1997).

Needle and syringe programs began illegally in Australia in 1986 (Wodak et al. 1987) but were soon adopted as government policy. As a consequence of the early and widespread introduction of needle and syringe exchange programs in Australia, impressive gains have been made, including the prevention of an estimated 2900 cases of HIV infection (Feachem 1996). Furthermore, this prevention measure has been very cost effective. It was estimated that the cost per life-year saved from syringe exchange was only A$350 (Feachem 1995). In 1998, it was clear that Australia had succeeded in the prevention of an epidemic—the prevalence of HIV remained less than 5% among injecting drug users. There is also evidence that the introduction of needle and syringe exchange programs has not caused an increase in drug use, which was one of the main objections to its introduction.

Switzerland and Germany are the only countries to have introduced syringe exchange schemes into their prison systems. In both countries no assaults with syringes have been reported to have occurred (Nelles, Dobler-Mikola & Kaufmann 1997; Stover 1996). The Swiss study found that the frequency of drug use and injection had remained stable and sharing had virtually ceased. There were no conversions to HIV, hepatitis B or hepatitis C during the study period.

Injecting rooms

Injecting rooms were established in Switzerland in 1987 with the intention of reducing the public nuisance caused by people injecting in public toilets and parks, as well as addressing public health problems such as HIV transmission and overdose. Injecting rooms are now generally well accepted by the Swiss public, although opposition arose when some injecting rooms were located in residential areas. Injecting rooms also operate in some German cities and the most impressive data come from Frankfurt where injecting rooms were introduced in 1991. Since that time the number of people dying from drug overdoses has steadily decreased each year. In contrast, the number of people suffering a similar fate in NSW has steadily risen (see Figure 6.1).

In 1997, the NSW parliament set up a Joint Select Committee to examine whether or not injecting rooms should be trialled or

Figure 6.1 Opiate deaths in New South Wales and Frankfurt

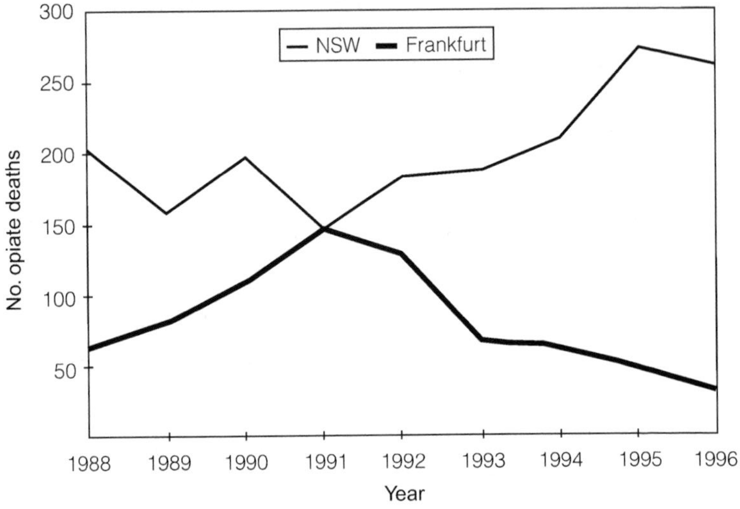

Sources: Joint Select Committee into Safe Injecting Rooms 1998; Lynskey & Hall 1998.

established, in response to a recommendation from the Wood Royal Commission into the NSW Police Service. The Committee was presented with an enormous amount of evidence, much of which was favourable (Joint Select Committee into Safe Injecting Rooms 1998). The Joint Select Committee decided against a trial of injecting rooms, although a trial would have provided the opportunity to answer many of the unknown questions about such an intervention. In fact, the NSW Drug Summit in May 1999 recommended that non government agencies should not be blocked from establishing injecting rooms.

The typical injecting room is small and has a 'sterile ambience'. It contains two or three tables where clients sit to prepare and inject their drugs. Injecting paraphernalia—such as needles and syringes, a candle, sterile water and spoons—are placed at each position at the tables where clients sit. There are paper towels, cotton pads, bandaids and rubbish bins nearby. The walls are usually tiled up to a height of approximately two metres and the table tops are made of stainless steel, which makes cleaning easier.

Heroin trials

Another strategy authorities are using to treat illicit heroin use is the provision of heroin under medical supervision. It is not a new treatment option as it has been operating in the United Kingdom since the 1960s. There was much political debate about a proposed ACT heroin trial in 1997. The Prime Minister decided at that time, against the advice of several committees, to veto the trial. Meanwhile, a number of trials have proceeded in Europe. The first trial was in Switzerland and it targeted injecting drug users who had failed other forms of drug treatment (Uchtenhagen et al. 1997). Over 1000 injecting drug users were studied over 18 months at 18 different locations, including a pilot study of prison inmates. Recruitment of patients, retention rate and compliance were better with the prescription of injectable heroin than with that of injectable morphine and methadone. Heroin caused fewer side effects than the other two drugs and improvements in physical and mental health occurred. The use of illicitly obtained heroin decreased rapidly. Housing situations of patients improved to the point where no one was homeless and the number unemployed fell from 44 to 20%. Income from illegal activities decreased dramatically from 59 to 10%, as did court convictions; a sizeable number of patients became drug free. There was an overall cost benefit per patient day of approximately A\$50, with most of the cost benefits coming from savings in criminal investigations and prison terms. Heroin trials have since commenced in Germany and the Netherlands.

Another procedure has received much media attention lately. It is the use of ultra rapid opiate detoxification with naltrexone. The procedure has been touted as a 'magic cure' as drug users become free of heroin in a brief time. It involves sedating a heroin-dependent person and inducing rapid withdrawal. After withdrawal, the patient is required to take naltrexone on a daily basis for 12 months. While doing so, heroin will have no effect on their body. However, there are risks involved in any procedure where anaesthetics are used. Also, if the person stops using naltrexone and commences using heroin again, they will have no tolerance and be at risk of overdosing and possibly dying. A number of research trials have commenced in Australia, the results of which will be known shortly.

Once a person has become drug free, they will usually need some form of rehabilitation so that they can join society again. Some drug users who use drugs for long periods lose everyday skills, such as dealing with rejection or disappointment without resorting to drugs. There are a number of places that rehabilitate drug users. Commonly known ones include Odyssey House or We Help Ourselves. Drug users live in these places for 12 to 18 months and are taught how to reintegrate into society. Residents learn skills such as assertiveness, problem solving, stress management and accepting personal responsibility. Most clients leave these centres after a few days or weeks, but those who persist seem to do very well.

CONCLUSION

This chapter has outlined the effects of the three different types of drugs: stimulants, depressants and hallucinogens. Illicit drug use (apart from cannabis) and injecting drug use are relatively uncommon in Australia. The characteristics of dependence and withdrawal from drugs were described. The chapter concluded with ways to respond to drug problems, including controversial measures such as injecting rooms, heroin trials and needle and syringe exchange programs in general society as well as in prison.

REFERENCES

Australian Institute of Health and Welfare (AIHW) (1999) *1998 National Drugs Strategy Household Survey*, Canberra: AIHW.

Ball, J.C. and Ross, A. (1991) *The Effectiveness of Methadone Maintenance Treatment: Patients, Programs, Services and Outcome*, New York: Springer-Verlage.

Blewett, N. (1987) *National Campaign Against Drug Abuse: Assumptions, Arguments and Aspirations*, NCADA Monograph Series No. 1, Canberra: AGPS.

Butler, T. (1997) 'Preliminary findings from the NSW Inmate Health Survey of the inmate population in the NSW correctional system', unpublished paper.

Caplehorn, J.R.M. and Ross, M.W. (1995) 'Methadone maintenance and the likelihood of risky needle-sharing', *International Journal of Addiction*, vol. 30, no. 6, pp. 685–98.

Collins, D. and Lapsley, H. (1996) *The Social Cost of Drug Abuse in Australia in 1988 and 1992*, National Drug Strategy Monograph Series No. 30, Canberra: AGPS.

Commonwealth Government of Australia (1996) *National Drug Strategy Household Survey Report*, Canberra: AGPS.

Dolan, K., Wodak, A. and Hall, W. (1998) 'Methadone maintenance treatment reduces heroin injection in NSW prisons', *Drug and Alcohol Review*, vol. 17, no. 2, pp. 153–58.

Dolan, K. and Wodak, A. (1996) 'An international review of methadone provision in prisons', *Addictions Research*, vol. 4, no. 1, pp. 85–97.

Feachem, R. (1995) *Valuing the Past . . . Investing in the Future: Evaluation of the National HIV/AIDS Strategy: 1993–94 to 1995–96*, Canberra: Commonwealth of Australia.

Gerstein, D. and Harwood, H. (eds) (1990) *Treating Drug Problems, Vol.1: A Study of the Evolution, Effectiveness, and Financing of Public and Private Drug Treatment Systems*, Washington: National Academy Press.

Gottheil, E., Sterling, R.C. and Weinstein, S.P. (1993) 'Diminished illicit drug use as a consequence of long-term methadone maintenance', *Journal of Addictive Diseases*, vol. 12, no. 4, p. 45.

Hubbard, R.L. and French, M.T. (1991) *New Perspectives on the Benefit–Cost and Cost-Effectiveness of Drug Abuse Treatment, Economic Costs, Cost-Effectiveness, Financing and Community-Based Drug Treatment*, National Institute on Drug Abuse Research Monograph Series, Rockville, MD: US Department of Health and Human Services National Institute on Drug Abuse, vol. 113, pp. 94–113.

Hubbard, R.L., Marsden, M.E., Rachal, J.V., Harwood, H.J., Cavanagh, E.R. and Ginsburg, H.M. (1989) *Drug Abuse Treatment: A National Study of Effectiveness*, Chapel Hill, NC: University of North Carolina Press.

Jacobs, M. and Fehr, K. (1987) *Drugs and Drug Abuse: A Reference Text*, 2nd edn, Toronto: Addiction Research Foundation.

Joint Select Committee into Safe Injecting Rooms (1998) *Report on the Establishment or Trial of Safe Injecting Rooms*, Sydney: Parliament of New South Wales.

Joseph, H. (1988) 'The criminal justice system and opiate addiction: A historical perspective', in Leukfeld, E. C. and Tims, F. (eds) *Compulsory Treatment of Drug Abuse: Research and Clinical Practice*, Research Monograph, Rockville: US Department of Health.

Kaplan, E.H. and O'Keefe, E. (1993) 'Let the needles do the talking! Evaluating the New Haven needle exchange', *Interfaces*, vol. 23, no. 1, pp. 7–26.

Lang, E. (1998) 'Drugs in society', in Hamilton, M., Kellehear, A. and Rumbold, G. (eds) *Drug Use in Australia: A Harm Minimisation Approach*, Melbourne: Oxford University Press, pp. 1–13.

Lurie, P. and Drucker, E. (1997) 'An opportunity lost: HIV infections associated with lack of a national needle-exchange programme in the USA', *Lancet*, no. 349, pp. 604–8.

Lurie, P., Reingold, A.L., Bowser, B., Chen, D., Foley, J., Guydish, J., Kahn, J.G., Lane, S., Sorensen, J., DeCarlo, P., Harris, N. and Jones, T.S. (1993) *The Public Health Impact of Needle Exchange Programs in the United States and Abroad: Summary, Conclusions and Recommendations*, Report prepared for the Centers for Disease Control and Prevention, September.

Lynskey, M. and Hall, W. (1998) *Jurisdictional Trends in Opioid Overdose Deaths, 1988–1996*, Sydney: NDARC.

Makkai, T. and McAllister, I. (1998) *Patterns of Drug Use in Australia 1985–1995*, Canberra: AGPS.

Manderson, D. (1993) *From Mr Sin to Mr Big*, Melbourne: Oxford University Press.

Metzger, D.S., Woody, G.E., McLellan, A.T., and O'Brien, C.P., (1993) 'HIV seroconversion among intravenous drug users in and out of treatment: An 18 month prospective follow up', *JAIDS*, vol. 6, no. 9, pp. 1049–55.

Nadelmann, E. (1993) 'Progressive legalizers, progressive prohibitionists and drug related harm', in Heather, N., Wodak, A., Drucker, E., Nadelmann, A. and O'Hare, P. (eds) *Psychoactive Drugs and Harm Reduction: From Faith to Science*, London: Whurr.

Nelles, J. Dobler-Mikola, A. and Kaufmann, B. (1997) 'Provision of syringes and prescription of heroin in prison: The Swiss experience in the prisons of Hindelbank and Oberschongrun', in Nelles, J. and Fuhrer, E. (eds) *Harm Reduction in Prisons*, Berne: European Publishers.

Nelles, J. and Harding, T. (1995) 'Preventing HIV transmission in prison: A tale of medical disobedience and Swiss pragmatism', *Lancet*, vol. 346, pp. 1507–8.

Newman R.G. and Whitehall W.B. (1979) 'Double-blind comparison of methadone and placebo maintenance treatments of narcotic addicts in Hong Kong', *Lancet*, 8 September, pp. 485–8.

Rydall, C.P. and Everingham, S.S. (1994) *Controlling Cocaine: Supply Versus Demand Programs*, Druley, P., Navaline, H., De Philippis, D., Stolley, P. and Abrutyne, E., August: *www.rand.org/publications/MR/MR331/mr331*

Single, E. and Rohl, T. (1997) *The National Drug Strategy: Mapping the Future*, Canberra: AGPS.

Stover, H. (1996) 'Harm reduction strategies in prisons', *Wiener Zeitschrift fur Suchtforschung*, vol. 19, nos 1–2, pp. 67–8.

Uchtenhagen, A., Gutzwiller, F., Dobler-Mikola, A. and Steffen, T. (1997) 'Programme for a medical prescription of narcotics: A synthesis of results', *European Addiction Research*, vol. 3, no. 5, pp. 160–3.

Ward, J., Mattick, R.P. and Hall, W. (1998) *Methadone Maintenance Treatment and Other Opioid Replacement Therapies*, Amsterdam: Hardwood Academic Publishers.

Wodak, A., Dolan, K., Imrie, A., Gold, J., Wolk, J., Whyte, B. and Cooper, D. (1987) 'Antibodies to the human immunodeficiency virus in needles and syringes used by intravenous drug abusers', *Medical Journal of Australia*, vol. 147, pp. 275–6.

COMMENTARY—CHAPTER 6

Richard Matthews

Kate Dolan has demonstrated that as drug use has a long history, so too does any attempt to modify drug use. Few societies have existed without using mood altering chemicals for ceremonial, religious or recreational purposes. Drugs used within a society have varied due to the vagaries of history. Alcohol, for example, which is accepted and widely used within our society, is anathema in other parts of the world, particularly in Islamic countries.

The harms that may arise from drug use can be divided into direct effects of the drug itself and effects related to the illegality of the drug. For example, liver damage secondary to alcohol abuse is clearly directly drug related. But a sexually transmitted disease in a sex worker who is dependent on heroin can be regarded as a secondary harm related to the illegality and consequent cost of the drug.

An additional complicating factor in drug and alcohol treatment is the widespread belief that misuse, in particular dependency, is in some way a moral failing. The labelling of individuals dependent on drugs as 'failures' is part of an entrenched judgemental culture within the general community, among many drug and alcohol workers and even among drug users themselves. The terminology and vernacular of the milieu further reinforces this belief. Expressions such as 'clean' and 'dirty' in relation to both drug use and urinalysis results are commonly used by clinicians and addicts. While the decision to use a particular drug for the first time is obviously voluntary, once dependency occurs, physiological changes mean that cessation and continued abstinence are not a simple matter of choice.

That drug and alcohol treatment has been overlaid with such moral judgements has meant the treatment field is driven with schisms which make the Byzantine church appear positively straightforward. Poorly evaluated 'feel-good' treatments, messianic-like cures, quackery and assorted 'God botherers' abound. In no other field of health care are so many patients placed in treatment because of an unquestioning belief in its efficacy. In no other field are so many poorly or non evaluated treatments continually supported by direct or indirect tax payer funding. In addition, the illegality of many drugs has resulted in uneasy partnerships being forged between law enforcement, the criminal justice system and treatment providers. There are often conflicts about court-mandated treatment programs, the requirements of probation and parole officers and the fears of clinicians in relation to patient confidentiality. For example, the view of many clinicians that a reduction in heroin use from three times daily to three times weekly is a positive treatment outcome is one not necessarily shared by the criminal justice system.

Nurses must have the skills to assess patients regarding the level of their drug use and the harm that it may be causing the individuals or those around them. In attempting to make this assessment it is useful to divide drugs into categories. A drug may be licit or illicit. Licit drugs may be further divided into prescribed and non prescribed. In relation to a particular drug a patient may be described as:

- a non user
- a user
- a misuser
- a dependent person.

As with other illnesses, the role of the clinician is to take an accurate history, perform a physical examination and arrange the appropriate investigations. These actions should lead to an accurate assessment of dependance, physical damage and risk.

The management plan should involve education and a discussion of risk and treatment options. Illegality is important but not central. Relapse is the norm. For example nicotine dependent patients suffer an average of five relapses before achieving abstinence.

Nurses working in other disciplines will frequently encounter drug misuse or dependency as an incidental finding: a narcotic addict may present with endocarditis. The businessman who suffers drug withdrawal after routine surgery and the elderly woman whose fractured femur occurred as a result of a surfeit of alcohol present different challenges. In these cases, accurate history taking is paramount and denial is frequent. It is important to establish good rapport in order to confront such denial.

These few examples show that a broad range of skills is required in drug and alcohol assessment and treatment. The ability to take an accurate history, perform a physical examination and formulate a management plan are the core competencies. A non-judgemental attitude, an understanding of harm minimisation and the ability to form a true therapeutic relationship are the attributes which lead to best practice.

7 Ageing

John Stevens & Julienne Onley

INTRODUCTION

> We are doomed historically to history, to the patient construction of
> discourses about discourses and to the task of hearing what has
> already been said (Foucault 1973, p. xvi).

Foucault observes that we are hearing what has already been said. The
authors of this chapter, during the researching and writing process,
were constantly questioning if this is in fact so. Are we, in our dealings
with the care of ageing people, turning a full circle—are we 'doomed
historically to history'? While perusing this chapter, we ask that our
readers also ponder that question.

Before the second half of the nineteenth century, both in Australia and overseas, older people did not exist as the social category
in the way we tend to perceive them today. Foucault (1965) and De
Beauvoir (1972) indicate no cultural mechanism or language existed
to distinguish socially the lame, lunatics, chronically ill, widows and
orphans, imbeciles—or the aged. They were identified not by their
infirmity but by their economy, that is, by their poverty. The unproductive were not able to sustain themselves and so placed a burden
on the economies of the communities in which they existed.

The social response to this threat to the economy saw the development of institutions to minimise the burden and, where possible,
maximise the profit from economic misfits. According to Norton
(1990), for example, by the start of the nineteenth century in England
there were over 4000 workhouses containing an unknown number of
able workers and 100 000 infirm residents, mostly older people, who

were unable to work (Longmate 1974; White 1978). No separate provision was made for the various categories of the infirm. Once inside the workhouse, married couples and families were separated. The inmates were often locked in, forced to wear drab uniforms, allowed no visitors or gifts and, of course, they had to work. Conditions fluctuated for inmates over the eighteenth and nineteenth centuries but few accounts indicate the workhouses to have been better than prisons for those committing the crime of becoming unproductive due to age, illness or destitution (Foucault 1965; White 1978).

From the arrival of the First Fleet in New South Wales there was a determination not to reproduce the European model of poor houses. During the mid to late nineteenth century, the Australian community entered into a period of enlightenment in the care of older people as it developed the language and the skills previously unavailable in society to recognise and accommodate older people in genuinely humane ways. Unlike the previous poor house and asylum culture, older people are now generally considered part of our community, not ostracised from it, hidden away and punished. Or are they?

As noted above, historically there has always been a fear of the burden that dependent, unproductive older people place on communities. Given some of the demographic predictions about our ageing population detailed later in this chapter, those fears are again being inflamed as we start the century. The challenges facing the community over its ageing population are the same as those faced by Australia over a century ago: balancing social expectations and human rights against what we are told we can afford. As we think about the future of caring for older people, the right balance could be achieved by underpinning the policies, discourse and actions with a consideration of how we would like to be judged by our counterparts one hundred years from now.

Following the presentation of the demographic factors facing our community, this chapter sets out to explore a brief history of aged care in Australia, which reminds us that many of the issues we think are unique surrounding the care of older people today have been with us for a long time. The chapter also explores some of the policies and actions, including that of residential care provision, being implemented today.

AUSTRALIA'S AGEING POPULATION

Rowland (1991) and Pollard and Pollard (1981) consider that a population is said to be ageing if the proportion of people over 65 years of age is increasing. According to that definition, Australia's population has been ageing since the early 1970s, a trend expected to continue for the next 50 years at least (AIHW 1998). The period 1976 to 2016 is expected to see significantly higher increases annually in the older population than for the overall population, the highest increase rates being among the very old (ABS 1996). In 1960, 5% (or 894 243) of the population was 65 years or older. Just 20 years ago, 1.3 million people, 9% of the population, were aged 65 and over. By 1996 this had increased to 2.2 million, representing 12% of the population. By 2016 this amount is projected to further increase to 16%, or 3.5 million people. The number of people aged 80 and over increased from one in six in 1976 to one in five in 1996 and will be one in four by 2016 (AIHW 1998).

While the older persons of the near future will never have been so healthy (Rowland 1991; Sax 1993), age is still a most accurate indicator of the need for health and welfare services (Fuchs 1984). It is interesting to note that 64% of older people living in the community rate their health as good, very good or excellent, although increasing age brings about a differential between men and women (AIHW 1998). The proportion reporting poor health in the 85 to 89 year age group is 27% for men, which is over double that for women (AIHW 1998).

Large cohorts of ageing people are expected to remain a factor in Australian population characteristics for many generations. Rowland (1991, p. 2) described this as 'population momentum'. Although declining mortality rates and migration have an effect on a population's trends, the major factor affecting the current demographic picture in Australia is fertility. There was a steep rise in birth rates between the late 1940s and early 1960s. This cohort has become known, affectionately, as the 'baby boomers'. Peaks and troughs are generally followed 65 years on by an equivalent peak or trough in the number of older people. The 'baby boomers' cohort is significant because there is a peak that lasts for nearly 20 years. The first of the baby boomers reach 'old age' (in this instance, defined as 65 years and over) just after 2010. This will be followed by a 'grey boom' that will last at least 20 years.

Another characteristic of Australia's ageing population is the growing disproportionate sex ratio. Women are living longer than men. Women born in the baby boom period have an average life expectancy of 80 years compared to men born in the same period, who have an average life expectancy approximately six years less than women—that is, 73.9 years (AIHW 1992). In the period 1994 to 1996, the life expectancy of Australians aged 65 was 19.6 years for women and

15.8 for men (AIHW 1998). Women make up over 60% of the population over 65 years and over and 75% of those are over 85 years. The outcome of this declining sex ratio is that there are and will continue to be many more older women than older men, more widows than widowers.

'In strictly demographic terms ageing is predominantly a female phenomenon and many of the problems associated with old age are disproportionately those of females' (Borowski & Hugo 1997, p. 32). Nay (1992), Sax (1993) and Speedy (1992) predict that old women are far more likely to experience financial hardships than older men because of the patriarchal nature of the society into which they have been born. Care of old people, therefore, will consist, as it does now, of mainly women caring for old women both at home and/or in institutions (Jones 1992).

THE HEALTH OF OLDER PEOPLE

One of the most common stereotypes about old age is that the elderly are unhealthy (Brower 1981; Brown 1977; Campbell 1971; Tuckman and Lorge 1953). In one respect the 1989–90 National Health Survey (AIHW 1992) might support this assumption. It revealed that the proportions of the population reporting one or more long-term conditions increased with age. Ninety-six per cent of people aged 75 years or over reported one or more disabling chronic conditions. The same pattern emerged for the reporting of recent illness. The same survey reported that, when asked, most old people saw themselves as healthy despite the presence of a number of infirmities (Alzheimer's Association 1993; Brody 1973). Elderly people perceive their health to be poorer if their independence and autonomy have been jeopardised (Vanclay et al. cited in Sax 1993). Fries (1984) and Rowland (1991) show that increasing average life expectancies advance the probability of acquiring a handicapping condition at the end of life, despite the better average health of the elderly in general (Fries 1984)—a phenomenon Fries has called 'compression of morbidity' (p. 36). Developing this concept, Jones (1992) believes that timely medical intervention, with its resulting longevity for many, is the most significant reason for the apparent rise in the prevalence of disability later in life.

The concept of 'compression of morbidity' is especially relevant when considering disability linked to dementia. Consistent with an increase in people living to older age, the number of people with dementia will increase. While estimates vary with definitions of dementia, it is estimated by the Australian Institute of Health and Welfare (AIHW) (1998) that 6% (134 800 people) of those over 65 years in Australia have dementia.

The understanding of preventative processes today will ensure that future cohorts of elderly people will age with better health than preceding cohorts. However, as Sax (1993, p. 58–9) suggests:

> [Many] . . . factors have the potential to improve health
> expectancies, but growth in the total population of old people will
> cause absolute increases in the numbers of elderly individuals with
> disabilities and handicaps. They will have a major impact on health
> and welfare systems.

While it is clear that disease and disability are common in older people according to the National Health Survey (AIHW 1998), this understanding must be balanced by the positive aspect that many older people are actually free of disease and disability. Many of those who are experiencing problems maintain positive and active lives. Whichever the case, all older people deserve equal treatment in health and welfare and ought not suffer age-based discrimination (McCallum 1997).

THE COST OF THE AGEING POPULATION

According to the AIHW (1998) the age of a population is a determinant of total health costs. In Australia it is estimated that in 1994, 35% of total health expenditure was for those over the age of 65 years, who represented just under 12% of the total population. In 1993–94, $11 billion of the total national health care expenditure of $31 billion was spent on people over the age of 65 years. The AIHW estimated that in 1994 health expenditure on people over 65 years was four times greater than for their younger counterparts. Over 31% of the total expenditure on pharmaceuticals was for those over the age of 65 years, 2.5 times higher than for younger persons in 1994. The AIHW predicts that people over 65 years will increase their use of the health care budget from its current one-third to a half by the year 2051 (AIHW 1997).

The AIHW notes that some of these figures can be termed a 'statistical illusion' depending on their interpretation. For example, included in the calculation of health care costs for older people are such aberrant items as the cost of food and accommodation. In addition, nursing home expenditure is the most expensive component of aged care accounting for 63% of the total $3.2 billion on specific aged care items in 1997. Further, approximately 13% of this sum is allocated to hostels, 21% for Home and Community Care (HACC) services (of which 1% is spent on assessment) and 2% is spent on community aid packages.

Is there a fear of the 'economic burden' of an ageing population directing policy? Economic statistics concerned with correlations with age make older people appear vulnerable. If the figures above do indeed provide compelling evidence, then our economy (and therefore the Australian community) should fear the ageing population. In reality, as McCallum and Geislhart (1996) state: 'costs have more to do with time from death than with time from birth'. Thus, population ageing per se has minor cost implications because, while it shifts the high cost period to later age groups, the period of time left until death is the significant cost factor, not peoples' chronological age groups. Overall it was estimated with reference to figures for 1994 that expenditure by older people was 1.9 times higher for medical services than expenditure for younger people. People over 65 years accounted for an expenditure 3.8 times higher than the health expenditure for those under 65 years. In 1994 the overall expenditure for older people was $4900 per person compared with $1300 for younger people, thereby increasing the years over which high costs are incurred. For instance, specific expenditure under the banner of aged care amounted to $3.2 billion in 1997. Most of this was spent on approximately 11% of the population over 65 years with severe disabilities receiving some form of care. This means that approximately 89% of people over 65 years made no claims on the amount designated as a specific aged care resource. While 63% of the aged care resource was spent specifically on people in nursing homes in 1995, the following data should be noted. Excluding those receiving respite (temporary) care, figures for 1995 showed over one-third stayed less than two months and the median length of stay was 356 days (AIHW 1995). While rigorously obtained figures are unavailable, anecdotal evidence suggests a figure above 90% died and was thus the reason for majority separations from nursing homes.

AIHW (1998) showed that in the period 1982–83 to 1994–95 Australian real health expenditure grew by 2.8% per person per year. Of this increase, 0.6% (one-fifth) per year was a result of the costs associated with an ageing population. The main contributing factors for growth in the use of health services by all people, but in particular older people, 'include greater expectations of being healthy and the introduction of new technologies' (AIHW 1997, p. 21).

In real terms there will be increased demands made for public, private and charitable services either as community assistance or as residential care. Measurements such as the dependency ratio are being used by authorities to create seemingly undeniable logical facts or propaganda—the 'spectre' of dependency. The dependency ratio, for example, is not the reliable indicator of the future of the public purse that we are led to believe. The dependency ratio makes assumptions that all people between 14 years and 64 years are financially productive. It omits to consider those people who have disabilities, the sick and the unemployed, parents and housekeepers and those in full-time education. It assumes that no older people are still employed, have private income or live independent of state support. It takes no account of older peoples' good health, increasing rates of pay and forced savings through superannuation (ABS 1996). As well, the contribution made by older people in voluntary unpaid work and caring for others is ignored.

Some economists, according to McCallum (1997), forecast a future impoverished state because of the ageing population unless public spending on older people is cut or eliminated altogether. But as Stevens (1999) suggests we need to focus on those who want to plan for an equitable future for all age groups rather than those looking for scapegoats.

COST VERSUS QUALITY CARE

Sax believed in 1990 that one of the probable ways in which the cost of the increase in services could be rendered less 'disturbing' may be through employing more nurses who can work autonomously and who can, due to their now comprehensive training, 'cover the services previously provided by a variety of different professions' (Franklin in Sax 1993, p. 7). However, a more recent dramatic push to reduce the costs of residential aged care has been to deregulate the aged care labour market. A deregulation of the aged care workforce has led to the reduction in the number of registered nurses and enrolled nurses by 28.5% between 1993–96 (2362 registered and 3974 enrolled nurses) (AIHW 1999). They have been replaced by another category of aged care worker, with considerably less training and skill, but who are cheaper to employ.

Indeed, the New Aged Care Strategy set in place by the Howard federal government in 1997 all but removed the term 'registered nurse' from the *Aged Care Act* lexicon. The new Act regulations regarding staffing requirements of aged care facilities stated that, for heavily dependent people, care was to be managed by a 'trained nurse'. This intiative provided an opportunity for aged care providers to interpret 'trained nurse' as either an enrolled nurse or certified assistant in nursing in order to economise on wages. The lobbying of peak professional and industrial nursing bodies to 'keep the nursing in nursing homes' encouraged the Minister for Health and Family Services to eventually define a 'trained nurse' to mean, in the majority of cases, a registered or enrolled nurse. This was later recognised in the requirements for only registered nurses or other appropriately qualified health professionals, such as medical practitioners and allied health practitioners, to carry out certain procedures for older residents of aged care facilities (Commonwealth Department of Health and Family Services 1998). If not for this nursing category review in the *Aged Care Act* in August 1998, registered and enrolled nurses would have all but lost their roles in residential and community aged care—roles initiated and maintained by nurses to the benefit of quality aged care and the profession for over 100 years. Stevens and Herbert (1997, p. 18) acknowledge:

> Such a loss of collective knowledge and experience of over 120 years
> would not only be intolerable in terms of quality care for older
> people but as an area for nursing to establish professional (in the true
> sense) practice like that of other professions such as medicine and law.

A BRIEF HISTORY OF THE ENLIGHTENED RATIONALISATION OF AGED CARE

How far have we come? In relatively recent times (the last 100 to 150 years) care of older people has been associated with nursing care. The concept of 'nursing homes' (more recently redefined as residential aged care facilities), for example, has only existed since the 1950s. In Australia as in most of the western world the coming together of nurses and older people in their special relationship has a very definite history (Stevens 1995). In Australia a period of enlightenment around the second half of the eighteenth century occurred in the care of older people. As noted in the introduction of this chapter, until this period older people in need had not emerged as a separate category in society. In Europe the poor houses and in Australia the state, regulated charitable asylums evolved to care for the indigent (and therefore at the time most of the poor aged) of society. Care amounted to little more than shelter and food and at times even that was scarce (Stevens

1995). Unlike Europe where poor houses were often depicted as social refuse deposits and inmates little better off than slaves, according to Norton (1990), Australia offered a more socially moral system of charitable and state run asylums up until the 1960s than could be found among the rest of the developed world. Yet until this period of enlightenment in the history of aged care in the mid 1800s, older people were not considered separately from the class of destitute. Records from the Benevolent Society's Pitt Street Asylum in Sydney for 1830 showed a typical aged demography for asylums of the time. Of the 140 permanent residents, 70% were over the age of 60 years, 20% were over 80 years and one resident was 105 years old. The asylums were, while not so in name, Australia's first formal residential aged care facilities.

The genesis of aged care and the nursing home (residential aged care facility) as we now conceive them in Australia evolved during the period between 1860 to the beginning of the twentieth century. This evolution was dominated by two phenomena. First, an explosion of social concern for the treatment specifically of older people in state care (as evidenced by the numerous Royal Commissions of Inquiry and media reporting); and second the resulting or coincidental arrival of the Nightingale trained nurses in 1868.

Numerous Commissions of Inquiry in the early 1860s polarised public debate regarding the treatment of inmates within the state funded charitable asylums. On one hand there were those who wanted to see significant improvements from the reported unhygienic, often brutal conditions those inmates universally experienced. On the other, the feeling was that inmates should consider themselves lucky there was any provision at all. One report from the Inspector of Public Charities exemplifies this attitude (identified today as an economic rationalist perhaps):

> that a portion of the large expenditure annually made on the
> charities might be avoided, could means be found for impressing
> upon the masses the advisability of exercising provident habits is self
> evident. The lesson however is one most difficult for government
> based on popular support to teach those of the community most
> inclined to squander their savings on self-indulgence, so long as they
> know they can, when adversity fall on them, cast themselves, through
> the charities on the public bounty (NSW Legislative Assembly
> 1887–88, p. 693).

Nonetheless improvements were promised but slow to follow. Not for want of commitment to improving the fate of older people but because there was no mechanism or tool to make it happen; that is, until, the arrival of the Nightingale trained nurses.

The arrival and evolution of the Nightingale trained nurses provided the community with the mechanism to develop skills and the language to allow older people to be recognised as a unique component of society. In New South Wales, parliament passed legislation in 1877 regulating the asylum labour force to ensure that the highly effective trained nurses were employed at all state and charitable institutions. Thus the Nightingale nurses were officially engaged in the care of older people and the infirm almost 17 years before similar legislation was passed concerning nurses' involvement with general, acute care hospitals.

The improvement brought to asylum inmates by the trained nurses was immediate and could be measured in humanitarian as well as economic outcomes, which will be discussed in more detail below. Yet debate continued along the same economic versus moral polemic as previously noted. Typical of the debates and discourse of the time, the Colonial Secretary, Sir Henry Parkes, was regularly challenged to justify to parliament the additional expenditure incurred by the employment of trained nurses.

In one reply (with which managers of residential aged care facilities and policy makers today might identify) Parkes stated:

> . . . public sentiment has changed as to the quality of relief to be afforded by these institutions. The inmates are more numerous and special duties not originally contemplated have been assigned to the asylums, giving them in some measure the appearance of general hospitals (Parkes in NSW Legislative Assembly 1887–88, p. 694)

Indeed, the Annual Report of the Director of Public Charities in 1892 noted that 43% of all New South Wales' patients were in asylum hospitals and the humanitarian improvements made at each asylum where the nurses were employed were also noted. General living conditions and hygiene improved, infectious diseases decreased and overall inmate morale improved. In addition, it was reported that it was costing £50 per year to care for patients in the general hospitals compared to £15 per year for those in the asylum hospitals.

The trained nurses were credited at the highest political and social levels for the improved care of older and infirm citizens as well as providing opportunity for the wider community by way of economic efficiencies in health care more generally. It became evident soon after their introduction that the skill of the nurses spawned a revolution affecting the care of older people that the medical profession (despite its arrival in Australia with the first fleet) on its own was unable to create. According to Stevens (1995), despite the obvious care quality and economic improvements introduced by the trained nurses the economic rationalist factions of the day argued (an example can be found NSW Legislative Assembly 1887–88, p. 695) that cheaper, less well trained employees could have achieved similar results.

The relationship between nurses and older people

The relationship between older people and nurses was no social accident but a carefully thought out solution to a community need. The relationship between the nursing profession and older people as it was in the late nineteenth century remains today under threat from political and economic pressures exerted at many levels of the community. For example, a minister of the crown is believed to have expressed surprise that nurses working in aged care are paid as much as their counterparts working in critical care areas, such as emergency departments. The minister is further believed to have inferred that most older residents in aged care facilities are not sick, just old, and do not need skilled nursing care. Given that the responsibility of government encompasses residential aged care provision, indeed, to repeat the question—how far have we really come?

Before addressing this question, and remembering the observations made earlier about the health of many older people, it must be stated that although many older people never need to move into residential aged care settings, there is a minority who do. And it is this minority, with their significant needs, who must not be abandoned or discriminated against by ill informed opinion driving or affecting policy, particularly regarding the qualifications and skills of their formal carers.

RESIDENTIAL AGED CARE

Are residents of aged care facilities merely 'old' or are they in fact sick? This chapter maintains that older people move into care because they are sick, not because they are living beyond a certain age. Their age is to an extent coincidental, although ageing changes and increasing longevity do contribute to frailty and disability. Qualified nurses do, as part of their role, care for the sick and, in the language of Sir Henry Parkes, the infirm. The major issues facing older people in need of care in residential settings clearly reveal that they require skilled nursing and medical care. Residential aged care facilities are health care establishments where skilled staff are required to provide appropriate care within a framework of quality standards. As they are the final 'home' for many residents, care is delivered in an environment that approximates as much as possible their own homes.

To support the argument for qualified and skilled nurses remaining the optimal workforce in residential aged care settings in both an operational and supervisory capacity, several issues relevant to older residents of aged care facilities will be expanded in this section. These issues are multi-systems disorders, earlier hospital discharge, high levels of acuity and associated care needs and responses to relocation to aged care facilities.

Multi-systems disorders

That Australia's population is ageing has already been established. This phenomenon, together with advances in technology and a growing awareness of the need to adapt lifestyles to achieve longevity, has created significant numbers of older people living with multi-systems disorders. The nature of these disorders often leads to disabilities that exacerbate both physical and mental frailty. One result is that many older people require extensive, skilled nursing management. Dementing disorders can also create a burden for older people, in particular those over 85 years of age. The progress of dementia itself leads to the necessity of specialised care and support. When dementia is concomitant with the multiple problems that are all too common in older age, such as osteoarthritis, osteoporosis, cardiac disease, chronic airways disease, strokes, neurological disorders such as Parkinson's disease, renal disease, liver failure and cancer, the resultant acuity requires highly skilled care (Onley 1997).

Earlier hospital discharge

Earlier hospital discharge, whether due to technological advances such as improved anaesthetics and surgical techniques, changes in hospital practices such as pre-admission work-ups or redefinition of readiness for discharge, creates concern for older residents of aged care facilities, as it does for those residing in the community. Duckett (1994, p. 87) suggests:

> The criticism of earlier hospital discharge occurs where community services are inadequate (or, at least, not forewarned) or the patient's family and friends have not participated in the decision about the appropriate time for discharge and have different expectations of the patient's health status on discharge.

In the same way as early discharge affects an older person's family and friends and community services, staff in residential aged care facilities receiving residents back to the facility, or newly admitting them, suffer if they have not benefited from consultation. The perception of staff in acute hospitals may or may not be that registered nurses working in aged care facilities will be able to provide sub-acute or, in some cases, acute care. The reality is that they can and do if they are well resourced with the requisite equipment, knowledge and skills. An obvious further requirement is that those registered nurses are in fact employed in residential aged care facilities supported by enrolled nurses. Facilities catering for residents with what are deemed 'low care' needs prior to an acute hospital stay and discharge may also be placed in the situation of receiving residents now needing a high level of care back to that facility. These will, in many cases, have no 24-hour registered nurse cover, and limited availability of enrolled nurses.

As Onley (1997, pp. 11–12) observes:

> Discharge one or two days post-surgical hip replacement or repair of a
> fractured neck of femur is not uncommon. This in itself demands a
> high level of skill and resources, but combined with the existence of
> the aforementioned concomitant disorders, with or without dementia,
> the required level of skills and resources, human, technological and
> other, rises markedly.

While data in Australia report shortening of length of stay in acute hospitals, although hospital patients in older age groups still stay longer than younger persons (AIHW 1998), the impact of older persons' status at discharge has not been widely examined in this country. Studies in the United States (Duggan 1994; Naylor 1990; Rantz 1990), however, reveal common themes emerging in the literature. In summary, these themes are: a greater acuity level, a need for more skilled staff hours, more deficits in activities of daily living, more nursing assistant time required, more rehabilitation services needed, increased deaths in nursing homes and increased provision of palliative care. In particular, Naylor's findings indicate that earlier hospital discharge leads to increased risk of re-hospitalisation, increased numbers of acute or emergency care visits by health professionals and that those discharged early require care more complex than that which most families can provide.

Complexity of care needs indicates the necessity for skilled nursing care. Most people do not choose to move into aged care facilities— they have to move from home because of increasing frailty or illness, disability and the inability to cope with resources available to them and their families in a home setting. They need and deserve support, skilled care and a high level of resources, that is, a high level of care consistent with their acuity. This care cannot be provided by unskilled carers in under-resourced environments.

Acuity levels

An Australian study conducted in a major Victorian teaching hospital indicates the high levels of acuity among older patients transferred to long term facilities (O'Hara et al. 1996). This study found that 30% of patients transferred to such facilities died within four days. The findings indicate a need for a high level of nursing care, including palliative care skills, in long term facilities that receive patients transferred from the acute care sector. Further evidence reveals a high incidence of functional decline among older people following periods of hospitalisation. One study suggests that the population under examination had become significantly more disabled three months following discharge and may have also been at risk of future exacerbated disability (Sager et al. 1996). This comment is supported by other researchers (Juneau 1996; Langer, Drinka & Voeks 1991) who report that skilled nursing care is required for mobility needs, activities of daily living, rehabilitation, and increased acuity demonstrated by complex disease interactions and early death following discharge from acute hospitals.

Following discharge to residential aged care facilities from acute hospitals, it is clear that under-trained carers will not be able to provide sophisticated nursing care and will only be able to furnish maintenance care. This will not relieve any pressure of readmission and repetitive use of general and specialised medical services in aged care facilities. However, the presence of specialty trained registered nurses in these facilities, together with the provision of equipment and other resources, will enable inter-service transition to be better managed and acute illness or the aftermath of surgery to be treated in surroundings which are familiar to residents and accessible to families (Onley 1997).

Relocation to aged care facilities

Relocation brings about its own difficulties with which older people have to contend; Young (1990) and Manion and Rantz (1995) describe relocation and its effects. Whether or not residents are admitted to aged care facilities via an acute care hospital or direct from home, they undergo the effects of relocation. They will be suffering from one or perhaps several chronic disease states, physical frailty, the cognitive dysfunction resulting from dementia, or a combination of all these. A transition, as do all life changes, can combine losses and opportunities. Enhancement of those factors that minimise personal loss while promoting personal satisfaction is a necessary imperative in the nursing care of older people changing their place of residence to live in an aged care facility. Major losses they experience include losses of youth, health, productivity and independence—difficult enough to face without the added burdens of illness and disability. Caring, empathetic individuals may certainly ease these losses, but the task of assisting newly admitted residents cope with them in the presence of illness is daunting for staff not specifically trained to do so.

Physiological and psychological disturbances can result from transfer from one environment to another, a phenomenon described as a relocation stress syndrome by Manion and Rantz (1995). The major characteristics of this syndrome include increased confusion in older people, anxiety, apprehension, depression and loneliness. Added to these characteristics are the underlying perceived losses of support systems, familiar environments and health status. Mikhail (1992) describes nursing staff as crucial to those suffering the effects of relocation—their presence is essential to recognise certain behaviours as manifestations of the psychological impact of moving to an aged care facility. Inappropriate medication may result from failure to recognise the effects of relocation, especially among those who suffer from dementia. Highly skilled nurses, working within a multi-disciplinary team, should be able to recognise the presence of relocation stress syndrome and manage it appropriately. Any management that avoids the use of hastily prescribed and/or requested medications will avoid the potential problems associated with injudicious use of drugs in older people.

CONCLUSION

Are we enlightened regarding care of older people? The issues raised in this chapter, most of which have been discussed, debated and argued with policy makers and bureaucrats, indicate that we are. These same issues have also been discussed at length with those who were charged by the Department of Health and Family Services in 1997–98 with re-engineering the Resident Classification Scale, with aged care industry organisation representatives, members of senate inquiry committees and others.

But who are the enlightened 'we'? Nurses are justifiably proud of the way they have consistently claimed and maintained that registered and enrolled nurses must remain in residential aged care and, in the broader perspective, in any other settings in which aged care is delivered: acute care hospitals, private and public; rehabilitation centres; palliative care units; community based health care organisations. Nurses involved in residential aged care are enlightened, and a considerable number of their colleagues working elsewhere who recognise their core business as aged care are also deserving of that descriptor. Consumers themselves recognise and have stated in many forums the need for skilled nursing care in residential aged care facilities—they too are enlightened.

But what of those who make policy? Are they enlightened? The future for aged care relies to a great extent on policy makers and their advisers. Their 'enlightenment' has historically been questionable, as outlined previously in this chapter. The Commonwealth government's aged care program that underpinned the *Aged Care Act 1997* has been reinforced in government publications since its inception. The aged care program's objectives are:

> To enhance the quality of life of older Australians through support for positive and healthy ageing and the provision of a cohesive framework of high quality and cost-effective care services for frail older people, people with disabilities, and their carers. (Australian National Audit Office 1998, pp. 11–12)

The Department of Health and Aged Care's objectives for the planning of the aged care program are, inter alia *Aged Care Act 1997* (Cwlth):

- to provide an open and clear planning process
- to identify community needs, particularly in respect of people with special needs, and
- to allocate places in a way that best meets the identified needs of the community.

These objectives, both of the aged care program and of the department responsible for administering it, appear enlightened, well founded even. However, has the translation into action seen a commitment to a responsive and informed residential aged care arena? Considering the issues raised in this chapter, and the expansion of those issues, the authors hesitate to answer that question in the affirmative.

Are we to return to the days of poor houses and asylums for the 'aged and infirm'? At least, as pointed out earlier in this chapter, the asylums were appropriately staffed by trained nurses and were economically viable. Therefore, if this was the result of fear driven policy and economic rationalism, perhaps the decisions leading to the staffing of the asylums could be described as responsive and informed—in fact, enlightened.

In Australia at present there are a range of residential aged care facilities which—if appropriately funded, resourced and staffed—will provide the best possible care for those older members of our community whose health status dictates that they need care. Those facilities that provide quality care will be rewarded by an accredited status and receive ongoing funding. But the proviso contained above in the small word 'if' is highly significant. If residential aged care facilities are facilitated by way of funding (and, indeed, mandated if that is necessary to cease misinterpretations by some employers) in their endeavours to provide the necessary care by appropriately qualified nurses, they will be able to meet the future with confidence. So too will their residents and potential residents.

The enlightenment, fostered and driven forward by nurses and supported by consumers, can continue, but only if care of the aged is allocated its fair share of resources and strategies, such as relevant clinically based research, are encouraged to ensure the most appropriate use of those resources. This will only result from informed policies, which are clearly, in a fiscal and strategic sense, the responsibility of government; that is, the responsibility of those within government and its bureaucracy who inform, develop and implement policy.

The use of the spectre of dependency in the aged and ageing section of the population could lead to fear of ageing and contempt of this so-called unproductive group among younger people. The fuelling of ill-informed debate, opinion and policy by fear tactics stemming from misunderstanding of the true nature of ageing could well lead this country back to days where residential aged care is provided in 'places of safety' (asylums in their true sense). There, care of the gentle, 'tender loving' variety could indeed be given, and fairly inexpensively. But would such environments, with the best will in the world, be able to foster and provide highly skilled nursing management and care, informed by research, and appropriate to the requirements of those with complex health needs? Are care arrangements for the aged driven by economics or health?

We have indeed come a long way since the mid 1880s, but unless we can maintain the momentum, nurses in aged care might well, although with enormous regret and reluctance, see the end of enlightenment.

REFERENCES

Alzheimer's Association of Australia (1993) 'Education and training on dementia issues and policy paper', North Ryde: Alzheimer's Association.

Australian Bureau of Statistics (ABS) (1996) *Projections of the Population of Australia, States and Territories, 1995–2051*, cat. no. 3222.0, Canberra: ABS.

Australian Institute of Health and Welfare (AIHW) (1992) *Australia's Health 1992*, Canberra: AIHW.

AIHW (1995), *Australia's Health 1995*, Canberra: AIHW.

AIHW (1997) *Aged Statistics*, Canberra: AIHW.

AIHW (1998) *Australia's Health 1998*, Canberra: AIHW.

AIHW (1999) *Nursing Labour Force 1998*, Canberra: AIHW, cat. no. HWL 14.

Australian National Audit Office (1998) *Audit Report No. 19, Performance Audit: The Planning of Aged Care: Department of Health and Aged Care*, Canberra: Australian National Audit Office

Borowski, A. and Hugo, G. (1997) 'Demographic trends and policy implications' in Borowski, A., Encel, S. and Ozanne, E. (eds) *Ageing and Social Policy in Australia*, Melbourne: Cambridge University Press.

Brody, S. (1973) 'Comprehensive health care for the elderly: An analysis', *The Gerontologist*, vol. 13, no. 4, pp. 412–18.

Brower, H.T. (1981) 'Social organisation and nurses' attitudes towards older persons', *Journal of Gerontological Nursing*, vol. 27, pp. 293–8.

Brown, I.M. (1977) *Nurses Attitudes Towards the Aged and Their Care*, Annual Report to the Gerontology Branch, USPHS.

Campbell, M.E. (1971) 'Study of the Attitudes of nursing personnel towards geriatric patients', *Nursing Research*, vol. 20, pp. 147–51.

Commonwealth of Australia (1998) *Portfolio Budget Statements 1998–99, Health and Family Services Portfolio, Budget Initiatives and Explanations of Appropriations 1997–98*, Budget Related Paper No. 1.8.

Commonwealth Department of Health and Family Services (CDHFS) (1998) *The Resident Classification Scale Training Workbook*, Canberra: CDHFS.

Cummins, C.J. (1971) *The Development of the Benevolent Asylum*, Sydney: NSW Department of Public Health.

De Beauvoir, S. (1972) *The Coming of Age*, New York: Putnam Publishers.

Duckett, S.J. (1994) 'Reform of Public Hospital Funding in Victoria', *Australian Studies in Health Service Administration No. 77*, Sydney: School of Health Services Management, University of NSW.

Duggan, J.M. (1994) 'Quality of care under casemix', *Medical Journal of Australia*, vol. 161, Supplement, pp. S18–20.

Foucault, M. (1965) *Folie et deraison. Histoire de la folie a l'age classique*, Paris: Plon.

Foucault, M. (1973) *The Birth of the Clinic*, New York: Pantheon.

Franklin, J. (1993) 'Crisis?' *The Bulletin of the Australian Psychological Society*, December, pp. 6–8.

Fries, J.F. (1984) 'The compression of morbidity: Miscellaneous comments about a theme', *The Gerontologist*, vol. 24, no. 4, pp. 354–9.

Fuchs, V. (1984) 'Though much is taken: Reflections on aging health and medical care', *Milbank Memorial Fund Quarterly*, vol. 62, no. 2, pp. 143–65.

Gibson, D., Mathur, S. and Racic, L. (eds) (1997) 'Older Australians at a glance', in *Australia's Health 1998*, Canberra: AIHW.

Jones, B. (1992) 'Chairman House of Representative Committee for Long Term Strategies', *Expectations of Life, Increasing the Options for the 21st Century*, Canberra: AGPS.

Juneau, B. (1996) 'Special issues in critical care gerontology', *Critical Care Nursing Quarterly*, vol. 19, no. 2, pp. 71–5.

Langer, E., Drinka, P.J., and Voeks, S. (1991) 'Readmissions and acuity in the nursing home: How will the nursing homes manage?', *Journal of Gerontological Nursing*, vol. 17, no. 7, pp. 15–19.

Longmate, N. (1974) *The Workhouse*, London: Temple Smith.

Manion, P.S. and Rantz, M.J. (1995) 'Relocation stress syndrome: A comprehensive plan for long-term care admissions', *Geriatric Nursing*, vol. 16, no. 3, pp. 108–12.

McCallum, J. (1997) 'Health and ageing: The last phase of the epidemiological transition' in Borowski, A., Encel, S. and Ozanne, E. (eds) *Ageing and Social Policy in Australia*, Melbourne: Cambridge University Press

McCallum, J. and Geiselhart, K. (1996) *Australia's New Aged*, Sydney: Allen & Unwin.

Mikhail, M.L. (1992) 'Psychological responses to relocation to a nursing home', *Journal of Gerontological Nursing*, vol. 18, no. 3, pp. 35–9.

Nay, R. (1992) 'An ageing society: Implications for nurses', in Gray, G. and Pratt, R. (eds) *Issues in Australian Nursing 3*, Melbourne: Churchill Livingstone.

Naylor, M.D. (1990) 'An example of a research grant application: Comprehensive discharge planning for the elderly', *Research in Nursing and Health*, Special feature, vol. 13, no. 5, pp. 327–47.

Norton, D. (1990) *The Age of Old Age*, London: Scutari Press.

NSW Legislative Assembly Votes and Proceedings (1887–88) *Inspector of Public Charities Annual Report 1887*, p. 4.

NSW Legislative Assembly Votes and Proceedings (1892) *Report of the Director of Charitable Institutions 1892*, vol. 8, p. 940.

NSW Legislative Assembly Votes and Proceedings (1894) *Annual Report of the Medical Advisor to the Government*, T.P. Anderson-Stuart 1894, vol. 5, p. 521.

NSW Legislative Assembly Votes and Proceedings (1896) *Report of the Select Committee on Pensions*, p. 5.

O'Hara, D., Hart, W., Robinson, M. and McDonald, I. (1996) 'Mortality soon after discharge from a major teaching hospital: Linking mortality and morbidity', *Journal of Quality in Clinical Practice*, vol. 16, no. 1, pp. 39–48.

Onley, J. (1997) 'The importance for the Australian community of maintaining a professional nursing presence in residential aged care facilities', *Geriaction*, vol. 15, no. 3, pp. 10–14.

Pollard, A.H. and Pollard, G.N. (1981) 'The demography of ageing in Australia' in Howe, A.L. (ed.) *Towards an Older Australia*, Brisbane: University of Queensland Press.

Rantz, M.J. (1990) 'Inadequate reimbursement for long-term care: The impact since hospital DRGs', *Nursing and Health Care*, vol. 11, no. 9, pp. 470–2.

Rowland, D.T. (1991) *Ageing in Australia*, Melbourne: Longman Cheshire.

Sager, M.A., Franke, T., Inouye, S.K., Landefeld, S., Morgan, T.M., Rudberg, M.A., Siebens, H. and Winograd, C.H. (1996) 'Functional outcomes of acute medical illness and hospitalization in older persons', *Archives of Internal Medicine*, vol. 156, no. 6, pp. 645–52.

Sax, S. (1990) *Health Care Choices and the Public Purse*, Sydney: Allen & Unwin.

Sax, S. (1993) *Ageing and Public Policy in Australia*, Sydney: Allen & Unwin.

Speedy, S. (1992) 'The contribution of feminist research', in Gray, G. and Pratt, R. (eds) *Towards a Discipline of Nursing*, Melbourne: Churchill-Livingstone.

Stevens, J.A. (1995) 'A career with old people: Do nurses care for it?' Unpublished PhD Thesis, Kensington: University of NSW.

Stevens, J. (1999) 'Ageism and economic fundamentalism', in Nay, R. and Garrat, S. (eds) *Nursing Older People: Issues and Innovations*, Sydney: Maclennan & Petty.

Stevens, J.A. and Herbert, J. (1997) *Ageism in Nursing Practice*, Canberra: Royal College of Nursing Australia.

Tuckman, J. and Lorge, I. (1953) 'Attitudes towards old people', *Journal of Social Psychology*, vol. 37, no. 3, pp. 249–60.

White, R. (1978) *Social Change and the Development of the Nursing Profession: A Study of Poor Law Nursing Service, 1848–1948*, London: Kimpton.

Young, H.M. (1990) 'The transition of relocation to a nursing home', *Holistic Nursing Practice*, vol. 4, no. 3, pp. 74–83.

ACTS OF PARLIAMENT

Aged Care Act 1997 (Cwlth), Canberra: Commonwealth Government, 1997, Part 2.2, Division 12, Section 12.2.

COMMENTARY—CHAPTER 7

Irene Stein

The strong historical backdrop provided by John Stevens and Julienne Onley positions the current aged care reforms for the reader. In this chapter the authors compare the care given to older people and lunatics in bygone Australian asylums with the care options being offered to older Australians today as a result of the *Aged Care Act 1997*. The authors assert that the issues of both social and political advancement since 1877 and the advent of the Nightingale nurses to care for older people are comparable to many of the issues currently being raised in contemporary aged care. Of interest is the fact that cost containment in caring for these aged people in 1877 held similar importance as it does today.

The comparison drawn between the early asylum times and contemporary practice in aged care is a compelling one and brings into sharp relief the current situation for many aged Australians. In particular, the level of enlightenment described in relation to aged care is contextualised in the presentation of the demographics of ageing, notably the advent and impact of the baby boomers on long term care demands and the subsequent potential impact of the reduction in fecundity. Improvements in technology that have led to an expectancy of a longer life span have failed, however, to address the vexing issue of an increase in the frequency of dementia. Relocation stress and issues related to gender bias are also considered in this context.

A further frame of reference is provided to us in relation to the real health care costs of the ageing population in the milieu of increasing levels of acuity. This increasing acuity necessitates the continuing employment of skilled practitioners in a variety of care settings. Of major significance is the need for skilled practitioners in facilities that provide accommodation and care for residents of both high and low care needs (formerly nursing homes and aged care hostels). To this end, the critical need for both registered and enrolled nurses

(Division 1 and Division 2 nurses) to be working in aged care facilities is emphasised by Stevens and Onley. This is argued in the environment of early discharge from acute care facilities and programs to both high and low care aged care facilities of frail, sick older people with complex care needs.

Stevens and Onley maintain that the existing climate of deregulation in aged care will encourage the reduction in the levels of skilled personnel working in aged care facilities. This reduction in skilled personnel is based on profit enhancement through the substitution of unskilled and cheaper staffing alternatives. This aspect of deregulation of the aged care arena must further increase the vulnerability of the aged population.

The authors conclude that the aged care reforms currently being implemented across Australia do not provide adequate or sustainable care for older Australians. This conclusion is predicated on issues such as the increase in multi-systems disorders among an ageing population and the earlier and often pre-emptory acute hospital discharge of older clients and resulting management problems. An appropriate deconstruction of the relevance and value of the dependency ration provided by the authors is important in terms of its impact on future policy formulation in aged care.

In brief, this chapter overviews the efficacy of the federal government's aged care reforms and questions the quality and the distance of the journey since the nineteenth century.

8 Extending life

Mary Chiarella

INTRODUCTION: DEFINING TERMS

When one is confronted by a chapter title such as 'Extending life' the immediate question that springs to mind is: extending life beyond what? Beyond a catastrophic event or illness which threatens to shorten that life? Beyond that which can normally be expected of a life? Beyond that which would naturally be described as a life?

Such questions demand that we define our terms. What do we mean when we talk about an extension of life? What do we mean when we talk about a life? Is *a* life different from the concept *of* life? And then, of course, if we are talking about extending life, what might we be avoiding? Death, or the process of dying? In some circumstances we may extend a life to give a person 'a few more good years'. In others it may well be that extending life only extends the process of dying, that the person whose life has been extended does not live in the sense of life as we may choose to define it, but rather dies over a longer period of time.

So, first of all let us examine what we mean by life, and how it might be extended. Biologists of course, would have no difficulty in defining life, at least at a cellular level. We can all recall in our early school biology lectures learning about the characteristics of living things. To be alive, scientifically, it could be argued that human organisms require adequate tissue perfusion for their major organs. By contrast, death has been defined as a permanent state of tissue anoxia (Mason & McCall Smith 1987, p. 209). But what does such a definition of life mean for nurses at the bedside? A person might be in a deep drug-induced coma and yet still have adequate tissue perfusion. By contrast, they may be suffering from a disease that renders their bodies unable to perform such functions unaided in the short term, but from which they will ultimately recover and lead a normal life. Is having adequately perfused tissues sufficient to suggest that a life is worth extending? Or even worth living? Yet if that person's tissue perfusion had not been artificially supported, the person's life would not have continued, despite the fact that one might return to an otherwise 'normal' life, whereas the other may continue in a deep coma and never recover.

Questions such as these have become far more prevalent over the years as mechanical methods of maintaining tissue perfusion have been developed. In the past, if the heart and/or lungs failed, adequate tissue perfusion would automatically cease. Although the individual cells of the body would continue to function until the remaining cellular oxygen supply was used up (Mason & McCall Smith 1987, p. 209), there would be nothing more that could be done. The person would have been dead, and they would have been clinically recognisably dead. Anyone who has nursed a dying patient and watched them closely will know how obvious the moment of death can be. This understanding that a person may not independently be able to sustain circulation or respiration and yet might be kept alive by artificial, scientific means required a re-definition of death. Death no longer necessarily occurred when a patient stopped breathing or their heart stopped beating—the brain would have to have suffered tissue anoxia for death to have occurred. As long ago as 1968 a committee of the Harvard Medical School published a set of criteria for determining when death had occurred, which recommended that death should be understood in terms of a 'permanently non-functioning brain' (Kearon 1995, pp. 25–6). The recognition of similar qualifying factors in Australia was evidenced by the definitions of death which were introduced into human tissue legislation (for example, *Human Tissue Act 1983* (NSW) s. 33). It was necessary to clarify this situation to enable perfused organs to be removed from patients who were recognised to be brain dead. As Justice Windeyer observed in *Mount Isa Mines Limited v Pusey* ((1970) 125 CLR 383, p. 395), 'Law march[es] with medicine but in the rear and limping a little'.

It is clear that with the introduction of chemical and electrical cardiac stimulation, increased knowledge of cellular physiology and artificial ventilation, tissue perfusion now need not necessarily cease. So life, thus scientifically defined, may be prolonged, if not indefinitely, at least for considerably longer than might previously have been anticipated. In another sphere, developments in public health can quite truly be said to have extended life in a most positive fashion. There is no doubt that over the past century many diseases such as smallpox and diphtheria which previously would not only have shortened life, but indeed might have ended life, have been well nigh eradicated.

PLACING A VALUE ON HUMAN LIFE

The problem is that acknowledgements of advances in science such as those described above do not answer questions about the value of the lives which have been extended. At this juncture it is important to acknowledge that there are those who would contend that it is not the role of other human beings to place a value on human lives. They would argue that a human life is sacrosanct because it is just that— a human life (Hall 1997; Wainwright 1996). Concerns have been expressed that questions about the value of human life are dangerous questions (Norris 1997), because they imply that some human lives may be more valuable than others—a 'slippery slope' argument that has overtones of Nazi Germany (see the very balanced discussion about this in Charlesworth 1989, pp. 63–4). But such questions have been asked for many years (Sir Thomas Moore 1516) and are now increasingly being asked, by parliamentarians, theologians, ethicists and health care professionals (examples are Kennedy 1996; Kuhse & Singer 1993; Muller 1997; Trnobranski 1996; Warnock 1996). Such questions are not necessarily the domain of health care professionals. Ian Kennedy made the observation in 1984 that 'the doctor has no greater expertise than the layman in dealing with ethical issues'.

Because the clinical possibility of extending life has increased, then questions about the utility of so doing must be addressed. To do otherwise would be to ignore the fact that human life is qualitatively so much more than the simple scientific fact of having one's tissues adequately perfused. Whether a life so extended is of value or not must depend on something more than just longevity. Max Charlesworth in his 1989 Boyer lectures offers a distinction between biological life and biographical life. He states that: 'Biological life is simply being physically alive and breathing; biographical life is the life of a human person with his or her own identity and history, relationships, ideals, aspirations and desires' (Charlesworth 1989, p. 56). Questions that now spring to mind are: how can we identify the value of a human life? Who is qualified to undertake such a process? If such a process is undertaken, what is the purpose of doing so? Is it to decide whose lives we ought to extend? Or to decide for how long a life ought to be extended? Or to determine criteria for allocating resources to life extension?

It would be naive to imagine that decisions are not continually made about extending (or not extending) life. They are made about patients of all ages (McInerney & Siebold 1995), and are made in all clinical settings from the ward or accident and emergency room (Reeves 1997) to the palliative care unit (Ogden 1997) and the nursing home (Wurzbach 1995). Such decisions may relate to whether or not to institute resuscitation (Herbert 1997); whether or not to institute therapeutic measures for someone who would otherwise die (Dunn 1998); whether or not to continue with life sustaining measures for someone who will die if such measures are discontinued (Haddad 1996); whether or not to provide treatment which may concomitantly shorten life (Dines 1995); or even whether or not to accede to a request to assist in ending life (Ogden 1996). It is probable the factors that would be taken into account when making such decisions would involve some form of assessment of the value of an individual's existing and potential life.

The English case of *Airedale NHS Trust v Bland* ((1993) 1 All ER 821) offers a prime example of such an assessment in the judgments of the House of Lords. This was the tragic story of Anthony Bland, a 21 year old man who had been in a persistent vegetative state (PVS) for three years after suffering severe crush injuries following the collapse of a stand at the Hillsborough stadium. Anthony Bland was breathing spontaneously; the only 'artificial' factor that was 'extending' his life was the artificial feeding which the nurses were providing via a naso-gastric tube. Clearly, if he was not fed, he would starve to death, as he was unable to feed himself due to his persistent vegetative condition. Perhaps even before discussing the decision of the court, it is noteworthy to state that Paul Wainwright has expressed an objection (valid, in my view, although the paper itself expresses a strong bias) to the use of the description 'vegetative'. He observes that:

> [I]t could be argued that we should question the acceptability of a label such as 'vegetative'. We have over a considerable period, gradually moved away from terms such as lunatic, imbecile, cretin, spastic, Mongol, mentally handicapped, epileptic, geriatric and so on, as labels for patients. This is not just one more example of the move towards political correctness, but rather recognises that such terms are dehumanising and demeaning, and have often become insults and terms of abuse. However, it now appears that we are content to refer to human beings as 'vegetative'; it is hard to think of a more dehumanising term (Wainwright 1996, p. 39).

The treating doctor and the parents sought a declaration from the court that the doctor:

> may lawfully discontinue all life-sustaining treatment and medical support and thereafter need not furnish medical treatment to [the defendant] except for the sole purpose of enabling [him] to end his life and die peacefully with the greatest dignity and the least of pain suffering and distress (*Airedale NHS Trust v Bland*, p. 859).

The declaration was granted in the High Court and confirmed by the Court of Appeal. The Official Solicitor, in his role as guardian ad litem, appealed to the House of Lords asking the broad question, 'In what circumstances, if ever, can those having a duty to feed an invalid lawfully stop doing so?' (*Airedale NHS Trust v Bland*, p. 859).

Their Lordships did not really seem to address this question directly, but did confirm the declaration granted by the High Court. For the purposes of our deliberations it is interesting to explore the reasoning behind the decision of their Lordships to discontinue prolonging the biological life of Bland. Some of the reasons for the decision to grant the declaration were undoubtedly derived from principles-based ethics. They asked the question, 'What was in the best interests of the patient?'. This is the question most readily associated with the principle of beneficence (to do good), but is, of course, difficult to answer when the patient is unable to experience anything at all (Wainwright 1996, p. 40). Lord Browne-Wilkinson inquired 'whether a responsible doctor has [already] reached a reasonable and bona fide belief that it is not [in the best interests of the patient to continue to receive intrusive medical care]' (*Airedale NHS Trust v Bland*, p. 883). Such an inquiry is most usually associated with the principle of non-maleficence (to do no harm) but it has been argued that to allow the man to die through lack of food and fluids could not possibly fall within such a remit (Wainwright 1996, p. 40). Other bases for the decision to discontinue feeding Bland were that there was no valid legal distinction between a decision to discontinue treatment and the decision not to commence it (per Lord Lowry, *Airedale NHS Trust v Bland*, p. 875); and the distinction that to cease to feed via a naso-gastric tube was an omission, rather than a positive act, such as a 'mercy-killing' would be (per Lord Mustill, *Airedale NHS Trust v Bland*, p. 885). Lord Goff addressed the competing principles of sanctity of life versus the principle of self-determination (*Airedale NHS Trust v Bland*, p. 866). However, this was fallacious on two counts: first, because the principle of sanctity of life was not upheld because at the end of the day, their Lordships gave permission for

Bland to die. Second, the principle of self-determination was never in question because it was expressly stated that Bland had never expressed an opinion on the matter (per Lord Goff, *Airedale NHS Trust v Bland*, p. 863). It can be seen that their Lordships found many different paths of legal reasoning to reach the same practical conclusion: that Bland's feeding should be discontinued. It is difficult to know whether any of the reasons advanced were indeed the real reason, since Bland was presumably as content or unfeeling alive as he would be dead. It was only the rest of the players in the tragedy who wished to act, and their well-being was not discussed as a potential or acceptable reason for such a decision.

Lord Browne Wilkinson concluded his judgment thus:

> [T]he conclusion I have reached will appear to some almost irrational. How can it be lawful to allow a person to die slowly, though painlessly, over a period of weeks from lack of food but unlawful to produce his immediate death by lethal injection, thereby saving his family from yet another ordeal to add to the tragedy that has already struck him. But it is undoubtedly the law and nothing I have said casts doubt upon the proposition that the doing of a positive act with the intention of ending life is and remains murder (*Airedale NHS Trust v Bland*, p. 884).

The judgments in the Bland case demonstrate the difficulty the law (and indeed society) has in coming to terms with the developments in medical science which enable us to extend life beyond an individual's potential, but then present us with the moral dilemmas of when to cease the assistance if the individual cannot continue to sustain themselves.

NURSES AND THEIR INVOLVEMENT

There is no doubt that nurses are significantly emotionally and practically involved in decisions to extend or not to extend life. Nurses as a group spend more time with patients than any other group of health care workers. They are the only group to provide a 24 hours a day, seven days a week permanent presence with patients in hospital, although it is acknowledged that other groups may provide a similar on-call service. In addition, since the majority of people today die in hospital (Bauman 1998, p. 224), nurses spend more time with more dying people than any other group and are probably more experienced and knowledgeable about the phenomenon of dying than any other group. Yet, despite these facts, they do not necessarily play a significant or even formal role in decisions to extend or not to extend life.

The decision to resuscitate a patient

Whether or not to resuscitate a patient is a matter of significant concern for nurses (Page & Meerabeau 1996; Poupolo 1997). Often on the ward the nurse may be the only health care professional when a patient suffers a cardiac, respiratory or cardio-respiratory arrest. In the absence of cardio-pulmonary resuscitation (CPR) the patient's life would undoubtedly cease, and thus the nurses present will be required to make the decision whether or not to perform CPR in order to attempt to extend the patient's life. It should be acknowledged that the performance of CPR does not by any means guarantee an extension of life. Over 50% of resuscitated patients die later because of neurological complications and over 20% of survivors suffer serious brain damage (Liss 1986). A study in the United Kingdom in 1995 revealed that only about 10 to 20% of those undergoing CPR in acute general hospitals live to be discharged (Wagg, Kinirons & Stewart 1995). But the difficulty for nurses is that the existence of the 10 to 20% weighs heavily on their sense of duty to extend life, and in the absence of a decision to the contrary, nurses do tend to resuscitate patients, regardless of diagnosis or prognosis. In a study of nurses' experiences of CPR, Page and Meerabeau reported that nurses 'find themselves not infrequently undertaking resuscitation procedures they deem to be highly inappropriate' (1996, p. 321). Although there are reports of nurse involvement in decision making about whether or not to institute CPR (Miles & Burke 1996), a recent major study (Poupolo 1997) revealed that despite the fact that a majority of nurses reported knowing the patients' preferences for CPR, nurses participated in discussions with patients and their physicians about CPR in only 13% of cases. This lack of involvement of nurses, the key players in immediate CPR institution, is reflected in certain policy documents. For example, *Dying with Dignity: Interim Guidelines on Management* (NSW Department of Health 1993), while canvassing the need for consultation, does not actually mention the word 'nurse' at all in the document and places the emphasis firmly on the physician–patient relationship. Such situations are untenable and cannot continue.

Since nurses most often have the primary responsibility for instituting CPR, they also need to have a primary involvement, with the patient and the physician, in the decision making process. It is obvious that decisions to attempt to extend or not to extend life by CPR have a direct impact on both the clinical actions of nurses and their emotional well-being (Dunn 1998; Herbert 1997; Page & Meerabeau 1996). Decisions to institute longer term resuscitation on a patient are probably a little less clear cut. When a patient is admitted, the clinical decision as to what treatment is to be instituted is a medical decision, although the nursing staff will need to be consulted regarding the resource implications of the treatment. Once the patient becomes a nursing, as well as a medical, responsibility the degree of nursing involvement in decision making increases. Decisions to institute new treatments that might further extend life in a patient who is already being nursed certainly require considerable nursing involvement, as the nurses will be very aware how the patient is tolerating existing treatments and may also be familiar with the patient's views on the process. Nurses often feel very distressed when life saving measures are undertaken on patients who have made express requests for these not to occur (Dunn 1998; Gustkey 1998; Wurzbach 1995).

Decisions to discontinue life-extending treatments

The important thing to remember about such decisions is that patients have a legal right to refuse treatment, which means that the impetus to discontinue treatment which might extend life may be patient, rather than clinician, driven. During the 1970s and 1980s the courts increasingly recognised patients' rights and patient autonomy in America, Canada, England and Australia. If a patient does not wish to be touched, they have a legal right not to be, which is protected by the tort of trespass to the person, specifically in civil actions in battery.

However, at common law, the requirement for a patient's consent to be touched can be overridden in an emergency, and also the person has to be mentally competent in order to give or withhold that consent. Because some terminally ill patients are no longer mentally able to withhold their consent at the time when they might wish to do so, statutory mechanisms have been developed in some Australian states in order to give legal effect to their wishes after they have ceased to be competent. South Australia pioneered this legislation with the *Natural Death Act 1983* (SA). Basically this statute enables people who are terminally ill to give advance notice in writing of their intent to refuse extraordinary life sustaining treatment. The statute defines both terminal illness and life sustaining treatment, and there has been some criticism of the legislation because of the narrowness of these definitions. Be that as it may, it was a bold attempt in its day, and was the first statute in Australia to attempt to give legal effect to the advance directives of the patient in relation to refusal of life sustaining treatment. The Northern Territory adopted a similar model in its *Natural Death Act 1988* (NT). South Australia now has a far more comprehensive and wide ranging piece of legislation, the *Consent to Medical Treatment and Palliative Care Act 1995* (SA).

Following the report of the Social Development Committee of the Victorian parliament entitled *Inquiry into Options for Dying with Dignity* (April 1987), the Victorian parliament passed a revolutionary piece of legislation in 1988, namely the *Medical Treatment Act 1988* (Vic.). The Act is much wider in its scope than the original South Australian legislation and establishes the right of a patient to register, by certificate, a refusal to accept medical treatment. It also enacts an offence of medical trespass and provides protection for doctors who act in reliance upon a certificate. Although the term 'medical treatment' is defined within the legislation, the right to refuse treatment is unqualified, and providing the patient understands what they are doing and they are competent to do so, the patient's right to refuse is the primary focus of the legislation. The provisions were further extended via the *Medical Treatment (Enduring Power of Attorney) Act 1990* (Vic.) to enable a person to appoint an agent to make the decision on the patient's behalf should the patient become incompetent. New South Wales has, as previously mentioned, its interim guidelines, *Dying with Dignity* (NSW Department of Health 1993), which only provide guidance for clinicians, rather than rights for terminally ill patients. However, the guidelines also canvass the use of advance directives, but there is no obligation on clinicians to observe them. Notwithstanding these limitations, patients in New South Wales still have their rights to refuse treatment under common law.

Where patients are no longer competent to refuse treatment and no advance awareness of their wishes are known, yet continuation of treatment may continue biological life, but not biographical life, such as for patients in a PVS, a number of different approaches have been taken. On many occasions, the decision to discontinue treatment which is considered to be futile is made locally without any anguish. As Charlesworth points out, even Pope Paul VI has accepted that upholding the sanctity of life is not an absolute duty (Charlesworth 1989, p. 60). This is particularly the case where the treatment might be to discontinue ventilating a patient or ceasing an infusion of inotropes which have maintained the cardiac output. The New South Wales guidelines make specific provision for such an eventuality.

In situations where the decision not to extend life might involve the withdrawal of food or fluids, the situation is less clear. Some clinicians have taken such questions to the court, as with the case of Bland, and others have sought the advice of ethics committees, but there is no doubt that decisions about these situations have also been made at clinical levels on a fairly regular basis. Once again, there is substantial evidence to suggest that nurses carry much of the burden of the consequences of these decisions. Although there seems to be a strong feeling among nurses that it is better to discontinue feeding than to prolong life indefinitely (Becker 1998; Goodhall 1997), some find these concepts unacceptable or distressing (Hall 1997; Wainwright 1996) and even hypocritical, in that they believe that such acts are in fact a form of 'slow euthanasia' (Ogden 1997). In addition, nursing patients until their death after food and fluids have been withdrawn can be very harrowing, as was graphically described in an article about a patient who took 20 days to die after the decision to withdraw food and fluids had been taken (Ohlenberg 1996). It is imperative that nurses are central to such decision making processes from the outset, as they will undoubtedly be central to the consequences of such decisions.

Decisions to accede to a request to assist in ending life

Here it is important to differentiate between a decision to discontinue treatment, which may end a life, and a decision to commit a positive act to either assist a person to end their own life (assisted suicide) or to end their life for them (voluntary euthanasia). Making a differentiation between voluntary and involuntary euthanasia is unhelpful, as committing a positive act to end someone's life without their request has to be some form of unlawful killing, and does not fit within the context of the modern debate on euthanasia. Thus, the definition of euthanasia used in this chapter is a positive act to end a person's life at that person's request and for that person's perceived benefit. The euthanasia debate is ongoing in Australia and has been well covered by other writers (an excellent recent example is Kerridge, Lowe & McPhee 1998, pp. 460–87) but it is a very important debate for nurses, because there can be no doubt that they will be directly involved with patient care before and after decisions are made about euthanasia.

The Northern Territory passed the first euthanasia legislation with the *Rights of the Terminally Ill Act 1995* (NT). This Act sought to define the processes by which a patient might seek assistance to end their life with voluntary euthanasia. However, despite the fact that nurses are so familiar with the fears, the pain, the moments of joy, the anxieties, the philosophising about the meaning of life and death—all the things which they have experienced so many times as they have nursed the dying—the legislation referred to nurses only in the definitions section under the types of health care provider to whom a doctor might give an instruction. And yet it is most likely the nurse to whom questions about euthanasia will be initially addressed. It is also likely to be to a nurse that an initial request for euthanasia would be made, and a nurse would probably explore that request with the patient to determine its origins and validity before either the patient or the nurse referred the matter to a doctor. Often in palliative care the nurse will have a close relationship not only with the patient, but also with the patient's family or significant others. Yet there is no suggestion in the legislation that the doctor should consult the patient's primary nurse for a second opinion on the patient's state of mind or the consequences of the request. It would have undoubtedly also fallen to the nurse to care for the patient during the 'cooling-off' period, the time after the request for assistance to end life had been made and the assistance was to be given. Nurses were not mentioned as key decision makers in any of the draft forms of euthanasia legislation that were produced in Australia, and yet the amount of responsibility which they would carry in practice is likely to be considerable.

Regarding the request for assistance, since all the draft legislation produced in Australia has envisaged that the assistance to die would take the form of a lethal dose of medication, it is clear that the formal request for a prescription must be to a medical practitioner, as only they would be able to prescribe the lethal dose of medication. However, in the long term, were euthanasia to be legalised, it is quite possible that the administration of the medication could be undertaken by a nurse. Indeed, if the nurse had a close relationship with the patient, they may be the most appropriate person to provide the assistance. There are numerous stories of nurses wanting to be present at the death of a very loved patient, or wanting to be the one to prepare the patient's body after death as a mark of respect and affection, as a final act (Knepfer & Johns 1989, pp. 223–4; Spiers 1997, pp. 76–81; Sullivan 1997, pp. 62–7).

There is a parallel with such a high level of nursing involvement, yet so little recognition of it in the abortion legislation. When the *Abortion Act 1966* (UK) was first passed, it was never imagined that an abortion would be performed by a nurse, because abortion was a surgical procedure in those days. Yet by 1981, when abortion began to be carried out by prostaglandin infusion, it was determined by the House of Lords that an abortion so induced was an abortion performed by a doctor so long as the doctor prescribed the drug and inserted the intra-cervical catheter. The fact that the nurse administered the prostaglandin and cared for the patient during the termination was not held to be significant as it was considered unreasonable to expect doctors to be present for the carrying out of every medication order which they made (*Royal College of Nursing (UK) v Department of Health and Social Security* [1981] AC (HL) 800). If this can occur in a situation where it was originally unimaginable that a nurse might be a key player in the process, how much more likely is it that the nurse could adopt such a role in a situation where the legislation makes specific provision for the doctor being able to instruct the nurse?

Whether or not a nurse ought to be involved in euthanasia is a matter for the nurse's own conscience, and any legislation must make provision for such a conscientious objection. However, it is imperative that nurses figure large both in the debate and in any future legislation, and must have the opportunity to be involved if they so wish. In the Netherlands, where euthanasia and assisted suicide are practised and not prosecuted, only the report of the Dutch State Commission on Euthanasia (Anonymous 1987; Smits 1993) mentioned the role of the nurse. The Royal Dutch Medical Association (RDMA) ignored the role of the nurse in its deliberations until 1988, when the RDMA and the Nurses' Association (known as Het Beterschap) presented joint guidelines on collaboration and the assignment of duties in cases of euthanasia and assisted suicide (Muller 1997, p. 425). These guidelines were revised again in 1991 by the RDMA and another nurses' association, New Union '91. These guidelines stated that nurses ought to be involved in the decision making process, because of their expertise and proximity to the patient, but the guidelines expressly stated that euthanasia and assisted suicide might only be administered by a doctor. Muller reported that on 7 October 1995 the High Court in the Netherlands found a Dutch nurse guilty of assisting with euthanasia, at the request of a friend and colleague who was suffering with AIDS. The patient's GP was present and advised the nurse throughout. No punishment was ordered for the nurse, but the judge made it clear that only doctors are allowed to assist (Muller 1997, p. 424). Muller's study to determine the extent of nurse involvement showed that specialist doctors involved nurses quite extensively in the decision making process about euthanasia and assisted suicide (only in 5% of cases did they not consult), whereas GPs did not consult in 45% of cases. However, despite the illegality of nurses' administration of euthanasia and assisted suicide, an unpublished study carried out by Onwuteaka-Philipsen and Van der Wal revealed that specialists allowed nurses to administer the lethal injections in 21% of cases (Muller 1997, p. 430).

Situations such as those described above are not uncommon for nurses. Nurses often undertake tasks that have been designated the domain of doctors for one reason or another, but which nurses are required to carry out because it is in the patient's best interest for them to perform it. This is just another situation where the role of the nurse needs to be recognised and legitimated.

CONCLUSION

Decisions to extend or not to extend life are complex and difficult, and require careful deliberation and much consultation and involvement of all key stakeholders. Nurses will always play a major role in the practicalities of such decisions, but have traditionally been excluded from the decision making process. There is a very pressing need for nurses to assert their right to be involved and visible in such decisions, both at policy and legislative levels.

REFERENCES

Anonymous (1987) 'Final report of the Dutch State Commission on euthanasia: An English summary', Bioethics, vol. 1, pp. 163–74.

Anonymous (1992) 'Guidelines RDMA and New Union '91 (in Dutch)', Medisch Contact, vol. 47, pp. 29–32.

Bauman, Z. (1998) 'Postmodern adventures of life and death' in Modernity, Medicine and Health: Medical Sociology Towards 2000, Scambler, G. and Higgs, P., (eds) London: Routledge.

Becker, M. (1998) 'Life and death: It's quality, not quantity', RN, vol. 61, no. 5, pp. 9–10.

Charlesworth, M. (1989) Life, Death, Genes and Ethics 1989: Boyer lectures, Sydney: ABC Books.

Day, L. (1995) 'Principle-based ethics and nurses' attitudes towards artificial feeding', Journal of Advanced Nursing, vol. 21, no. 2, pp. 295–8.

Dines, A. (1995) 'Does the distinction between killing and letting die justify some forms of euthanasia?' Journal of Advanced Nursing, vol. 21, no. 5, pp. 911–16.

Dunn, M.C. (1998) 'Knowledge helps health care professionals deal with ethical dilemmas', American Operating Room Nurses Journal, vol. 67, no. 3, pp. 658–61.

Goodhall, L. (1997) 'Tube feeding dilemmas: can artificial nutrition and hydration be legally or ethically withheld or withdrawn?', Journal of Advanced Nursing, vol. 25, no. 2, pp. 217–22.

Gustkey, K. (1998) 'Weighing the rights of those who are terminally ill', RN, vol. 61, no. 1, p. 9.

Haddad, A.M. (1996) 'Ethics in action', *RN*, vol. 59, no. 5, pp. 21–4.

Hall, J.K. (1997) 'Speak up! Killing, not caring', *RN*, vol. 60, no. 6, p. 68.

Herbert, C.L. (1997) '"To be or not to be"—an ethical debate on the not-for-resuscitation (NFR) status', *Journal of Clinical Nursing*, vol. 6, no. 2, pp. 99–105.

Hunt, G. (ed.) (1994) *Ethical Issues in Nursing*, London: Routledge.

Kearon, K. (1995) *Medical Ethics: An Introduction*, Dublin: Twenty-third Publications.

Kennedy, L. (1996) 'Dignity in death', *Nursing Standards*, vol. 11, no. 11, p. 19.

Kerridge, I., Lowe, M. and McPhee, J. (1998) *Ethics and Law for the Health Professions*, Sydney: Social Science Press.

Knepfer, G. and Johns, C. (1989) *Nursing for Life*, Sydney: Pan Books.

Kuhse, H. and Singer, P. (1993) 'Voluntary euthanasia and the nurse: An Australian survey', *International Journal of Nursing Studies*, vol. 30, no. 4, pp. 311–22.

Liss, H.P. (1986) 'A history of resuscitation', *Annals of Emergency Medicine*, vol. 15, pp. 65–72.

Mason, J.K. and McCall Smith, R.A. (1987) *Law and Medical Ethics*, London: Butterworths.

McInerney, F. and Siebold, C. (1995) 'Nurses' definitions of and attitudes towards euthanasia', *Journal of Advanced Nursing*, vol. 22, no. 1, pp. 171–82.

Miles, J. and Burke, L. (1996) 'Nurses' views of the decision not to resuscitate a patient', *Nursing Standards*, vol. 10, no. 22, pp. 33–8.

Muller, M. (1997) 'The role of the nurse in active euthanasia and physician-assisted suicide', *Journal of Advanced Nursing*, vol. 26, no. 2 pp. 424–30.

Norris, P. (1997) 'Never say die', *Nursing Standards*, vol. 11, no. 21, p. 21.

NSW Deparment of Health (1993) *Dying with Dignity: Interim Guidelines on Management*, Sydney: State Health Publication No. (HPA) 93-33.

Ogden, R. (1996) 'AIDS, euthanasia and nursing', *Nursing Standards*, vol. 10, no. 36, pp. 49–51.

Ogden, R. (1997) 'An open secret', *Nursing Standards*, vol. 11, no. 52, pp. 24–5.

Ohlenberg, E. (1996) 'We withdrew nutrition-not care', *Registered Nurse*, vol. 59, no. 5, pp. 36–40.

Page, S. and Meerabeau, L. (1996) 'Nurses' accounts of cardiopulmonary resuscitation', *Journal of Advanced Nursing*, vol. 24, no. 2, pp. 317–25.

Poupolo, A.L. (1997) 'Preferences for cardiopulmonary resuscitation', *Image Journal of Nursing Scholarship*, vol. 29, no. 3, pp. 229–35.

Reeves, K. (1997) 'Euthanasia, assisted suicide, and the right to die', *Journal of Emergency Nursing*, vol. 23, no. 5, pp. 393–4.

Royal College of Nursing (1991) *Living Wills: Guidance for Nurses*, London: Royal College of Nursing.

Smits, M.J. (1993) 'The role of nurses in euthanasia' (in Dutch), *Tijdschrift voor Verpleegkundigen*, TVZ 47, 764–7.

Spiers, H. (1997) 'A night to remember' in Taham, A. (ed.) *From the Heart: True Stories by Australian Nurses*, Sydney: Lothian Books.

Staunton, P.J. and Whyburn, R. (1997) *Nursing and the Law*, 4th edn, Sydney: WB Saunders/Bailliere Tindall.

Sullivan, E.C. (1997) 'Into this good night', in Tattam, A. (ed.) *From the Heart: True Stories by Australian Nurses*, Sydney: Lothian Books.

Trnobranski, P. (1996) 'The decision to prolong life: Ethical perspectives of a clinical dilemma', *Journal of Clinical Nursing*, vol. 5, no. 4, pp. 233–40.

Wagg, A., Kinirons, M. and Stewart, K. (1995) 'Cardiopulmonary resuscitation: Doctors and nurses expect too much', *Journal of Royal College of Physicians*, vol. 29, no. 1, pp. 20–4.

Wainwright, P. (1996) 'Persistent vegetative state: Ethical issues for nursing', *Nursing Standards*, vol. 11, no. 9 pp. 39–44.

Warnock, Lady (1996) 'Dying wishes', *Nursing Standards*, vol. 10, no. 52, p. 18.

Wurzbach, M.E. (1995) 'Long-term care nurses' moral convictions', *Journal of Advanced Nursing*, vol. 21, no. 6, pp. 1059–64.

COMMENTARY—CHAPTER 8

Michael Walsh

In her contribution, Mary Chiarella provides us with a clear and incisive discussion of the question of extending life and the involvement nurses ought to have in the process of decision making.

The chapter begins by defining life and death in the light of technological advances. Both are important as they indicate how the whole discussion of life extension is cast in a new light which makes us face new decisions. Max Charlesworth's distinction between biological life and biographical life helps to focus the treatment of the value of human life. Ultimately what we decide in terms of treatments and the effort put into them will be influenced by some 'assessment of the value of an individual's existing and potential life'.

To illustrate, Chiarella examines the case of Anthony Bland and its eventual resolution by the House of Lords. The quote from Lord Browne-Wilkinson highlights both the matter of life and its quality, and the legal and ethical dilemma of the common distinction between killing and allowing to die. This distinction could have been further discussed, but it is well rehearsed in the literature, and may have distracted from the point Chiarella is making, namely the involvement of nurses in the decisions to extend or not extend life.

It is here that Chiarella makes her strongest contribution. Nurses are so deeply involved in the care of dying patients that it is incomprehensible that they are left out of the process of decision making. The fact that the New South Wales interim guidelines, *Dying with Dignity*, do not mention the word 'nurse' in the entire document ought to be considered an outrage by the nurses of this state. Nurses are involved in the continuing care of patients and often involved in attempts to resuscitate. They are, therefore, often in the best position to know the wishes of many of the patients. As Chiarella points out, in the future they may also be involved in administration of lethal medication if the law should change to allow euthanasia. It is imperative that nurses be fully involved in the wider social debate and also in the processes of decision making.

PART III

Health care delivery

9 Clinical information systems

Dianne Ayres & Lyn Perks

INTRODUCTION

This chapter will discuss the role of information systems in health care. It will focus on systems at the point-of-care to assist nurses, doctors and allied health professionals (clinicians) with information to support clinical practice, education and research. The 'point-of-care' refers to any location where a clinician delivers health care to a patient and may be in a hospital, clinic or GP's office. The emphasis of this chapter is about the internet delivering decision support information and point-of-care systems to generate orders, results, charts, clinical pathways, reports and discharge summaries.

Health care is a turbulent market, with bed and hospital closures, decreases in length of stay, a dynamic and highly educated clinician workforce, care delivery methods that are constantly remodelled to achieve best practice, and health care technology that is ever changing. The public health system is also evolving as a competitive market: hospitals in rural and remote areas need incentives to attract and retain professional staff; major teaching hospitals market their services to attract tertiary referrals from other health enterprises. Effective information systems are needed to support current trends and to maintain a leading edge. The environment is complex and one in which health care organisations function to ensure that the goals of the information systems support the goals of the corporate missions and organisational strategies. Information drives corporate efficiency and productivity and must be managed, nurtured, preserved and, most importantly, used effectively (Commonwealth of Australia 1997).

Information resources should be considered as the real business assets while information technology is the enabler that helps create, store and provide access to that resource.

Information is a critical resource in health care as in other industries. Doctors, nurses and allied health professionals rely on information to make decisions that affect the health outcomes of their patients. Timely, accurate and reliable information could mean the difference between life and death, an accurate or erroneous diagnosis, early intervention of therapy or a prolonged and costly stay in hospital. Health is an information intensive industry and, because of the paucity of information technology in health care, clinicians must currently manage most of this information manually. This is made more difficult in an environment where patient acuity in hospitals is higher because of a reduction in patient length of stay. Without compromising the quality of care, clinicians must do more with less and learn to work smarter. Information technology is the only realistic means of managing information more efficiently. It is the enabler in integrating information across multiple care settings, reducing duplication and errors of omission, transcription and interpretation, and providing timely information in the right location. In other industries, information technology decreases production costs; in health the gains are more qualitative. These include better patient outcomes as technology such as magnetic resonance imaging (MRI) and positron emission tomography (PET) scanners and knowledge databases all contribute to more accurate diagnoses and enhanced decision making.

The following section focuses on the internet as a means of providing information and communications tools to support clinical practice, education and research, which will enhance and support decision making and clinical care processes. Providing information using this medium is complementary to a point-of-care information system that delivers order entry, results reporting, clinical pathways/care plans, assessment, charting, medical alerts, notes and discharge summaries for clinical care management. This section also briefly describes the genesis of the internet and the development of the world wide web as the user interface to today's internet. Much has been written about the internet that cannot be covered in this chapter. We encourage you to read an excellent text called *A Guide to Medical Informatics, the Internet and Telemedicine* by Enrico Coiera (1997) for a detailed insight into informatics, including the internet and the world wide web.

THE INTERNET PHENOMENON

At the beginning of the twenty-first century, the information revolution with its advances in information and communications technology places no geographical boundaries on the distribution of data and knowledge. This global information infrastructure has opened up a world of communications that has no limitations.

The internet is one concept of distributed computing that has revolutionised the communication of information. The concept of distributed computing (using PCs and servers) means that users have flexibility and openness in features and functions that are quite unlike the centralised mainframe computer and dumb terminal of the past (Orfali, Harkey & Edwards 1994, p. 11). The internet is a 'network of networks' first developed in the late 1960s by the Department of Defense in the United States to distribute information, safe guarding it from the threat of nuclear attack. The system was then known as ARPANET (Advanced Research Projects Agency Network). The expansion of the internet was slow until 1985, when the merging of the NSFNET (National Science Foundation Network) and ARPANET opened up communications to universities and private corporations, forming the internet.

Over the past five years the internet has grown steadily to more than 40 000 networks electronically connecting over 40 countries. An Australia-based internet research group, www.consult, which conducts frequent online surveys, cited two million regular users in Australia by mid year 1998 and 327 million worldwide (Marzbani 1998). The Internet Industry Almanac predicted in 1998 that Australia would have eight million users in the year 2000. While internet utilisation statistics vary quite considerably from source to source it is clear that the rapid growth rate of the internet is a remarkable phenomenon. As electronic commerce (e-commerce), online shopping and electronic banking gain the confidence of users there is no doubt this will contribute to the growth of the internet.

The desire to transmit different kinds of media other than text resulted in the development of the world wide web (the web) in 1989. The web is a sub-set of the internet with its own servers and a browser as its initial interface. The web has significant characteristics that make it easy to navigate and search the internet. Users can access multi-media including documents, graphics, animated images, photographs, audio and video. Hypertext is another important feature of the web, providing the means to navigate within a document or to other hyperlinked documents in any location on the internet.

The development of the world wide web has seen the internet capture the attention of the world like no other communications medium and has evolved to be the subject of magazines, a myriad of books and journals and numerous television programs that enthusiastically advocate particular web sites.

THE INTERNET AS A TOOL OF MODERN HEALTH CARE

The development of the web as a graphical interface to the internet is one of the greatest information technologies to come out of the 1990s (La France 1997, p. 1). Its flexibility and intuitive features enable information to be easily distributed to the point-of-care—where the focus needs to be in terms of providing quality information. The primary emphasis in today's health care system is to provide cost effective quality care that is equitable and integrated across the continuum of health care providers. Clinicians are the health care system's most expensive resource and the quality and quantity of information that is available in the right location to provide decision support is less than optimal. Information contributes to knowledge and clinical wisdom. It is therefore one of the most important resources for clinicians to achieve effective health outcomes for their patients. The internet offers a cost effective solution to provide quality decision support information using best practice standards and a communications infrastructure to enhance clinician productivity at the point-of-care.

The internet is an inviting communications medium because the web provides single point access to information, a diversity of content and sophisticated search engines. These features make access to information easy, even for novice users. The concept of ease of access to information is appealing to clinicians who work in a system where information is widely dispersed across a variety of entities. In the paper/manual system, documents are expensive to publish and require storage space. Large volumes of documents must be distributed to appropriate staff throughout the health system. Inevitably, documents do not always reach the staff who 'need to know' and communication of information is a well recognised problem within large organisations. The advantage of internet technology is that the user can 'pull' information rather than it being 'pushed' by the publisher (Coiera 1997, p. 253; Telleen 1997, p. 1). In other words, users can access the information that they *want* and need, rather than what they are sent 'just in case' they *might* need to read it.

Electronic communication via e-mail, news groups, mailing lists, bulletin boards and chat lines enable clinicians to consult with colleagues on specific topics or problems via the internet. For clinicians from rural and remote areas, this technology can minimise the sense of professional isolation and eliminate the disconnection created by distance.

The internet provides access to a vast range of health information from numerous sources. However, the difficulty for the user is the ability to locate the necessary information and validate the quality and credibility of that information. The need for quality information to support clinical practice, education and research was recognised by NSW Department of Health and resulted in the creation of a web site that provides access to a credible range of accredited information resources available in one location at *www.clininfo.health.nsw.gov.au*. This web site is known as Clinical Information Access.

The Clinical Information Access Project

The electronic universe encompasses a large area of information resources enabling clinicians to tap the brains and collective wisdom of thousands, perhaps millions, of clinical colleagues worldwide. The Clinical Information Access Project (CIAP) web site provides information services via online knowledge databases such as Medline, Cinahl, MIMS, and Cochrane Collaboration which are used to enhance decision making and support clinical practice. Traditionally, accessing these knowledge databases required a visit to the library, but now this information is accessible at the point-of-care. Information that is available where and when it is needed has the potential to improve the quality of patient care, reduce costs of health care, improve the efficiency of clinicians and the effectiveness of the care provided. This view is supported by Klein et al. (1997, p. 489) who assert that effectiveness of care is influenced by diagnostic and treatment decisions based on the availability of substantive current information from the most recent literature found in online knowledge databases. A number of studies on the effect of literature searching have shown that the information has changed the way particular clinical conditions are managed, contributed to better informed decisions and resulted in improved quality of care (Klein et al. 1997, p. 490). Aspects of care that were influenced included diagnosis, medications prescribed, length of stay and patient education. These findings are consistent with CIAP, which has the following information objectives:

- to ensure that health professionals have reliable and rapid access, 24 hours a day, to relevant information necessary to support care delivery
- to promote best practice by providing online access to clinical information from national and international sources
- to provide access to quality information from a single source at the point-of-care, which will contribute to better informed decisions and improve the quality of care
- to provide a source of accredited information to support research that will contribute to the delivery of evidence based health care
- to eliminate distance as a barrier to information access for clinicians in rural and remote locations
- to create an information culture that encourages health professionals to use information technology as an essential tool of modern medicine
  to promote consumer involvement in their own health care by providing the general public with rapid, convenient access to accredited health information resources.

The CIAP web site provides all health professionals in the New South Wales public health system with access to a wide range of information. A survey of 2700 clinicians determined the web content and all requests have been delivered including the following:

- Medline and CINAHL with over 12 million citations and links to 30 full text journal articles
- the full Cochrane Library with over 500 evidence based reviews
- PsycINFO linked to ten full text journal articles
- MIMS for prescription decision support
  HealthStar
- therapeutic guidelines
- Harrison's *Medical Textbook*
  Poisindex, Toxpoints, Martindale's and Drugdex from the Micromedex databases
- interactive ECG
- online tutorials
- policies, procedures, protocols, clinical practice guidelines and clinical pathways from contributing Area Health Services
- Department of Health policies and guidelines
- links to international and national clinical web sites
- listservers—an e-mail facility that enables communications between users with similar interests.

This web site is constantly evolving as new sources of information are identified and procured. All health professionals have the opportunity to contribute documents that adhere to the publishing guidelines posted on the CIAP web site.

Clinical representatives were established in each Area Health Service to liaise with the project team and assist in communications, marketing and education. This network of clinicians was an essential element in the success of the project and the enthusiastic uptake of the internet, particularly in rural and remote areas. Barriers to the uptake of the internet included: low penetration of PCs in clinical areas; inadequate telecommunications infrastructure; negative attitude to internet access; inadequate information technology resources; speed of the internet. Addressing these barriers is evolutionary and fundamentally reliant on funds becoming available to improve the status quo. The increasing demand for efficient delivery of information using the internet is already emerging as the catalyst to overcome the barriers. The telecommunications infrastructure will be upgraded as newer communications technologies are adopted and PCs will be purchased as many new information systems are implemented to meet a myriad of business needs. Attitude to internet access will improve as an information culture evolves and there is a dependence on the internet to deliver information in this new global information economy.

This web site has already contributed to improved communications across the continuum of care by enabling access to all health care providers, bridged the communications gap between hospitals, general practice and community services and reduced the sense of professional isolation experienced by rural and remote practitioners. Clinicians have formed their own information management committees to direct clinical initiatives; listservers (e-mail groups) are being used to communicate and disseminate information across the state; and several NSW Department of Health committees clinicians, including a collaborative committee with the health education sector and general practice, are driving clinical information reforms. An information culture has been born and will continue to thrive as clinicians adopt information technology as a tool of modern health care.

THE EVOLUTION OF POINT-OF-CARE SYSTEMS

Clinical information systems were first developed in the United States in the 1970s. Large mainframe computers enabled information technology staff at major medical centres to begin unifying all patient information to a single source. These initiatives required the investment of millions of dollars each year to develop and maintain the programs. Due to the unique configurations at each of these centres and the technology focus of the era, these systems were rarely reproduced elsewhere. The functionality they provided then (and still do today) was known by the generally accepted term of 'results reporting'. It included demographics and alerts and provided an excellent level of security for patient information.

The second phase of clinical system development included 'order entry' as well as the results reporting modules. Software companies wrote these systems in the late 1970s and early 1980s. As PCs were not widely used at that time, development was still conducted on mainframe or mini-computers. The primary purpose of this generation of clinical systems was to streamline ordering functions and reduce administrative costs. Ordering tests enabled patients to be scheduled directly and created efficiencies by removing paper forms, facilitating the printing of labels for blood collection and sorting tests to provide a logical collection route for laboratory technicians. These staff savings were repeated in ordering diets, radiology tests and pharmacy. All costs could also be linked to a single patient 'identifier'.

When these systems were developed, industrial engineers intended that the person initiating the orders should enter their own requests. However, in the United States and Canada, this was not the case. At that time, physicians were not familiar with information technology. They had never typed and therefore continued to write orders into the traditional charts. These orders were then transcribed by ward clerks or nurses, and checked for accuracy by nurses. Although many steps were removed from the ordering process and ancillary departments achieved efficiencies, nurses bore the clerical load by undertaking a task that they had not been previously required to perform.

There were financial benefits of this type of system, but none that could be directly attributed to reducing the clinician's workload. While a great deal of expectation was built up during implementation, this type of system failed to gain broad acceptance by clinicians involved in direct patient care. A notable exception to this rule involved the implementation of a patient care system at Veterans' Affairs Hospitals in Australia. Order entry, results reporting and patient scheduling functionality has been operational since 1990. At the Concord Repatriation and General Hospital in New South Wales, clinicians enter their own orders and have declared many benefits from the system (Soar, Ayres & Van der Weegen 1993, p. 373). This application is currently being replaced by a PC-based system.

A lesson for the learning

About 1990, development began on the new generation of clinical systems in the United States and Canada. Clinicians were also becoming more knowledgeable about new technology and what it could, and should, deliver for them. At the same time, a state health department in Australia tendered a clinical information system. In the bid to implement stable and tested technology, a system of the early 1980s genre was chosen. This was ultimately rejected by more informed clinicians and the application was decommissioned in 1995. Some studies have been undertaken to determine how this well-intentioned project could have gone so wrong. In fact, it did not deliver benefits for clinicians and failed to consider emerging clinician groups focusing on health informatics and new technology.

In 1996 the NSW Health Department Clinical Systems Reference Group, consisting of 50 clinicians throughout the state, developed a benefits methodology and determined the type of clinical systems that should be implemented in hospitals over the coming decade. This 'Clinical Information Requirements Report' (Clinical Systems Reference Group 1996) is published on the internet on the Clinical Information Access Project web site at *www.clininfo.health.nsw.gov.au/reports*.

THE STATUS OF CLINICAL SYSTEMS IN AUSTRALIA

There are few clinical systems implemented in Australia that can provide the functionality defined in the *Clinical Information Requirements Report*. True integration of diverse delivery mechanisms and resources cannot be achieved with systems that are focused on departmental solutions and are generally oriented only to inpatient care. In South Australia, four renal units from different hospitals have implemented an application that links all patients across hospitals and provides all information on dialysis and renal transplants undertaken in the state. In Western Australia, an application was selected in 1993 to provide results reporting and order entry capabilities for clinicians. This is implemented in nine hospitals in Perth and the greater metropolitan area and is currently being upgraded to include decision support capabilities such as drug interaction and allergy checking.

There are a limited number of applications in the New South Wales public system for integrated care management. The most notable is the Critical Care Information System at the New Children's Hospital at Westmead in Sydney. Several teaching hospitals are also in the process of implementing sophisticated systems that will provide integrated patient information, including outpatient data.

THE NEXT STEP

The need for a clinical information systems foundation that supports care delivery is a high priority for many clinicians. The question is, how will clinicians reach where they strive to be? There is no simple answer but it is mandatory that nurses know the essential elements of a robust information system to ensure that wise investments in information technology are made and nurses' information needs are met. Given the financial constraints of all Australian health systems, it is unwise to proceed down a path that will not enable us to achieve long term goals.

Technology can offer several ways to retrieve and view information. These solutions can look 'modern' by using graphical user interfaces (GUI) and web browser 'front-ends'. However, they are limited in what they can offer clinicians in the long term. It is therefore imperative that nurses know the questions that must be asked and understand the logical building blocks for clinical systems of the decades ahead.

Information systems with the complexities that will be described require millions of dollars annually to research and develop. They cannot be developed successfully without sufficient resources. However, without such complexities, decision support capabilities cannot be achieved. As decision support is one of the primary benefits recognised by clinicians, it must always be in the forefront when defining user requirements and evaluating proposals.

Much publicity has been given to the notion of the electronic medical record (EMR). We believe that the claim of totally electronic records made by some application vendors is not achievable in the short to medium term. The cost of technology, complete removal of paper from hospitals and the cultural backgrounds of traditional medical practitioners are issues that will only be resolved in the course of time. Many clinicians also have differing ideas of what an electronic medical record should contain.

It is advisable that system requirements and functionality be defined on a modular basis. This will enable clinicians to describe and understand what they need and want, rather than aiming for an undefined electronic medical record which may never be realised. When selecting an application, it is wise to determine if the vendor has the capability of providing this functionality—that is, electronic medical records—even though they may not be required for the initial implementation. By ensuring that sufficient vendor funds are directed to application research and development, a growth path is ensured, hence maximising investment.

The functionality of point-of-care clinical systems in the future will incorporate the components described in the following section. They are represented below in a logical order to provide a phased implementation approach. Each component provides a sound basis for the next phase.

PHASE 1: RESULTS REPORTING

This will enable test results and reports from all online service departments to be viewed in one location with a single log on. Clinicians will be able to customise the way they view results and display patient trends. Information will also be viewable across episodes of care to facilitate diagnosis and responses to treatment. To achieve this longitudinal view, all patient information will be stored in a single repository or database.

Medical alerts

An essential feature of this functionality is the ability to capture and display medical alerts such as allergies and risk factors. This will ensure that a decision support system can be provided in the 'order management' implementation phase.

Discharge summary

This facility enables a summary of patient admission history to be transmitted to other health care providers via fax, e-mail or letter. The template can be defined to include relevant information for each practitioner and should be flexible to allow the inclusion of additional information as further modules are implemented.

Reporting

This facility provides for the generation of standard and user defined reports to assist in unit management and clinical decision making. Each subsequent module will contain additional features that require further report definition.

Clinical databases and references

Clinical information resources, such as Medline, the Cochrane Collaboration, and clinical practice guidelines complement this core information and support decision making at the point-of-care. Additional documentation, such as protocols, policies and procedures specific to each organisation, should also be available and maintained online.

PHASE 2: ORDER MANAGEMENT

Order management will enable clinicians to order tests, procedures and services electronically. The orders will be received instantaneously in departments such as diagnostic imaging, laboratory, allied health, food and nutrition services, pharmacy and other ancillary departments. This module provides order tracking and duplicate order checking and can realise many benefits in ancillary departments, previously described in this chapter.

To gain clinician compliance, the order system must be rules based and provide clinical decision support. This functionality will ensure that the order is appropriate for each patient, will provide supporting information and suggest alternative measures as approved by each site. Several major software vendors have decision support rule sets available, but each hospital must determine if they are applicable to its clinical practice protocols.

Patient history

Templates for recording patient history are provided by major vendors. These should also support ongoing review at any time during the episode of care.

PHASE 3: CLINICAL PATHWAYS

Clinical pathways are predefined sets of orders. Therefore, order management must be implemented prior to commencing this initiative. These pathways enable all activities within an episode of care to be sequenced according to a predetermined plan. The development of these routines should be evidence based for a diagnosis related group. However, as many patients have multiple diagnoses, primary and secondary pathways must be accommodated to ensure that adequate staffing resources are allocated to care for these patients.

There is a great deal of debate around clinical pathways. Many clinicians claim that they are 'cookbook' medicine. However, if there is variance in clinicians' methods of treatment, each clinician can define their own pathway. As evidence is gathered over time, outcomes analysis can be performed. This will lead to refinement of best practice or evidence based outcomes.

Patient acuity pathways

Patient acuity is one of the most contentious issues for nursing managers and one of the most challenging pathways for application developers to design and implement. To gain maximum efficiencies, this measurement should be invoked as a secondary pathway when they are initiated, or as required after admission. The pathway can then add the hours of care required for specific patients, transfer these to the rostering system and enable care to be accurately costed.

Clinical documentation

As the clinical pathway provides a 'best practice' plan for all patient care, variances from that path should be the only documentation required. This module would provide a facility for all care providers to document such variances for subsequent outcomes analysis. In areas where clinical pathways are not initiated, this module would allow for a narrative report to be entered. Ideally this would be achieved through the use of a template to retrieve relevant data from disparate sources and prompt clinicians to use the predefined reporting standard.

PHASE 4: CHARTING

This supports the processes of documenting clinical observations and provides alerts for abnormal ranges. Ideally this information should be entered at the point-of-care, reducing duplication of effort and should be achieved through the use of mobile computer technology.

The technology

All current information systems are developed to run on PCs. Large capacity computers are used to manage the application and databases of clinical information but these are transparent to users. Expert staff of clinical information but these are transparent to users. Expert staff are required to service and maintain each of these critical elements. The rate of change for technology is also rapid. For example, PCs and laptop computers are superceded every few months by new and faster models. Application developers create information systems to run on the latest technology—it would not be a sound decision for them to do otherwise. However, this means that health services must review capital acquisition policies and implement innovative ways to stay abreast of the technology and application investments.

CONCLUSION

As information management becomes an integral part of patient care, information services departments are developing funding models such as memoranda of understanding (MOU) and service level agreements (SLA). The challenge for clinicians and business managers will be to understand the 'total cost of ownership' and apportion divisional funds to ensure that they can keep pace with the inevitable changes ahead of us all.

REFERENCES

Clinical Systems Reference Group (1996) 'Clinical information requirements report', NSW Health: *www.clininfo.health.nsw.gov.au/reports*

Coiera, E. (1997) *Guide to Medical Informatics, the Internet and Telemedicine*, London: Chapman & Hall Medical.

Commonwealth of Australia (1997) 'The global information economy: The way ahead': *www.dist.gov.au/itt/golds/*

Internet Industry Almanac (1998): *www.consultco.com.au/pub_press_6.shtml*

Klein, M.S., Ross, F.V., Adams, D.L. and Gilbert, C.M. (1997) 'Effect of on-line literature searching on length of stay and patient care costs', *Academic Medicine*, vol. 6, no. 69, pp. 489–95.

La France, S. (1997) 'Web technology and healthcare: Breaking boundaries', *HIMSS '97 The Big Picture Proceedings*, San Diego, vol. 4, pp. 3–11.

Marzbani, R. (1998) 'Fifth www.consult Australian on-line survey completed': *http://www.consultco.com.au/pub_press_6.shtml*

Orfali, R., Harkey, D. and Edwards, J. (1994) *Essential Client Server Survival Guide*, New York: John Wiley & Sons.

Soar, J., Ayres, D. and Van der Weegen, L. (1993) 'Achieving change and altering behaviour through direct doctor use of a hospital information system for order communications', *Australian Health Review*, vol. 16, no. 4, pp. 371–82.

Southon, F.C., Sauer, C. and Grant, C.N. (1997) 'Information technology in complex health services: Organisational impediments to successful technology transfer and diffusion', *Journal of the American Medical Informatics Association*, vol. 4, no. 2, pp. 112–24.

Telleen, S.L. (1997) 'Intranet paradigm': *http://ip.com/html_docs/info/Intraparadigm.html*

COMMENTARY—CHAPTER 9

Jeffrey Soar

This chapter addresses a fundamental challenge for information professionals in health care—how do we help our organisations become knowledge based and take advantage of the internet revolution?

The future health care world will be populated by knowledge workers who will employ evidence based approaches to planning and evaluation of services. Organisations will need to invest in knowledge warehouses and in the means for rapid access. Evidence based health services will target consumer need and specific interventions will be selected on knowledge of their research base.

The internet already links the world's major repositories of research. The challenge is in integrating these into planning and care delivery. Point-of-care information systems will provide a means of integrating patient information with the world's evidence repositories. Information processing in hospitals and other facilities is still largely manual including the exchange of information such as orders, results, care plans and medication plans via paper-based systems.

There are many providers involved with the care of an individual patient. Linkages between GPs, community pharmacies, independent midwives and other specialists and providers within hospitals are still either paper-based or non-existent. The chapter reports on the exciting Clinical Information Access Project (CIAP) for internet information access. The next steps will need to be exchange of patient information. Pilots of such sharing between primary, secondary and community-based carers through intranets/extranets are already underway in New Zealand and there are plans for a national intranet to link all providers. Expected benefits include better tracking of child immunisations. Any carer can readily check if the child in front of them is fully up-to-date with 'well-child' checks and immunisations. The same technology could allow checks for alerts, medication interactions, for laboratory or other diagnostic results thus reducing unnecessary examinations or tests while providing access to the most up-to-date patient clinical history.

The internet could be history's most rapidly adopted and pervasive technology. It offers a common user interface that links knowledge repositories, reducing the need for duplication of data in other databases.

10 Health care as a market place

Debbie Picone

INTRODUCTION

At the time of writing this chapter, state and territory political leaders are calling for an urgent national inquiry into the Australian health care system. This is somewhat incongruous with the reality that Australia is one of the healthiest countries in the world as measured by declining death rates, increasing life expectancy and, for the majority of Australians, ready access to some form of health care (AIHW 1998a). So why is there such concern at this time?

Perhaps the main trigger is the fact that health has been undergoing rationalisation over the last decade in an effort to ensure greater efficiencies in the system to meet increasing demand and associated increases in health expenditure. The demands on the health system are extreme as a result of new and costly clinical treatments, changing social demography, rising consumer expectations and an ageing population. The health system's capacity to manage this demand is limited.

Rationalisation has led to claims that the system is becoming too much like a business focusing on costs and outputs. There is also a prevailing view that only more money will solve all the perceived problems of the health care system. The fundamental tension is to reconcile potentially unlimited health needs and wants with finite resources and to ensure that existing resources are being used effectively.

This chapter will critique the current commentary around 'health as a market place' and offer recommendations relating to improving the effectiveness and quality of the health care system. It will do this through analysing the structure and administration of health services in Australia, health services funding, expenditure, access and usage as well as the quality and effectiveness of hospital services. This critique is informed by my 25 years experience as a clinician, clinician manager and senior health executive. All but two of these years have been involved in the daily reality of providing health services to people who attend the acute public sector for care and to date involves responsibility for ensuring the provision of health care to an extremely socially and economically disadvantaged group of people: approximately 6700 on a daily basis.

Some would say that this chapter describes a biomedical model of health. I agree. It describes a model that focuses on an illness system, rather than on a health system. For this reason my analysis of the health care system and proposed future directions for health care delivery is limited. While the approaches I have suggested are necess-ary, timely and desirable, they provide only a part of the solution and would best be considered as a starting point to encourage broader deliberation. This chapter has, because of word constraints, omitted discussion of issues relating to health promotion, illness and disability prevention and most importantly the issue of health inequalities and the links between health and equity.

The NSW Minister for Health recently announced the estab-lishment of a NSW Health Council (Healthcover 1999). This Council has been established to advise on setting the strategic directions for a health system into the next century (Healthcover 1999), not a small job by any means. Of course, the Minister has every reason to be concerned that despite record levels of state funding, demands on the system are growing faster than government can provide if the funding level remains the same in terms of percentage of gross domestic product (GDP). Demands have been put down to several issues. Australian projections state that there will be 3.5 million people over the age of 65 by 2016, representing 16% of the population. By the same year, it is estimated that one person in four will be over the age of 80 (AIHW 1998b). The increased use of technology, increased turnover of patients, trend towards day only surgery, increased expec-tations and number of patients with multiple problems also affect cost. On the other hand, more sophisticated technology has enabled signif-icantly improved management of certain illnesses through accurate investigation and therapeutic treatments. But the disadvantage of this has been that these occur mainly in the acute end of the health/illness spectrum, leaving groups such as the chronically ill, the disabled and those in remote areas, missing out in terms of funding and access to adequate services.

As well as the additional demands on the public system because of advances in medical science and higher consumer expectations, there has been a decline in people holding private health insurance, mainly due to the increasing gap between insurance rebates and medical bills. The current Commonwealth–state funding arrangements create significant barriers and disincentives to a more efficient and effective allocation of resources. For example, the Commonwealth funds GPs, while the states fund hospitals, thereby fragmenting care across the various boundaries between hospitals and community (Healthcover 1999), since costs require shifting between sectors. When a patient from a nursing home (also funded by the Commonwealth) is transferred into an emergency department costs immediately shift without the funds necessarily following. The widening gap between the respective demands on the public and private systems may also be an indicator of a system coming under considerable strain.

For all of these reasons it is no wonder that regular media coverage reports a health care system in crisis (Duckett 1999). We also read regularly about medical clinicians, nurses, politicians, consumers and other commentators claiming particular problems in the health care system. These include overcrowded hospitals and emergency services, long waiting lists and, more recently, the decline in private health care insurance, all used as evidence of the impending collapse of the health care system.

This troubled and often anxious rhetoric at many levels is not new, however, having continued unabated for the past 20 years, making health one of our foremost examples of public policy set around a media circus, rather than providing solutions. It is a near epic tale of federal/state rivalries, of Premiers' Conferences, vested interests and state marginal seats all perpetuating assertions of collapsing private/public sectors and a system in chaos. While this is played out, the media capitalise on the drama through their reporting of patients' deaths as a sign of the systemic deterioration in the quality of public health services.

But is our health care system really in terminal crisis? Is it about to break down? Has the time now arrived to reform the structure, delivery and funding of our health care system? After all, whether health care is in crisis or not, many opportunities certainly exist to better manage demand, control costs and improve health outcomes so that we have a system which is appropriate for the future.

THE STRUCTURE AND SCOPE OF THE AUSTRALIAN HEALTH CARE SYSTEM

There is no doubt that health is one of the nation's largest industries and as such may be identified as a business. It employs 400 000 health professionals, maintains 1130 hospitals and 2822 residential aged care facilities (AIHW 1999) and provides revenue for several hundred Australian and international suppliers of health products. Health services expenditure in Australia was estimated to be $47.3 billion in 1997–98 or 8.4% of the nation's GDP. Per person, expenditure on health services was $2536 in 1997–98 (AIHW 1999).

Currently the health system is controlled by scores of government bodies and boards, by Australian and overseas corporations, and by hundreds of industry organisations and pressure groups. It provides employment for groups as diverse as university academics, lawyers, journalists and marketing firms. But it is in the allocation of services that health is most unlike a market place. In the main it allocates services on the basis of need rather than capacity to pay, although inequities still exist in the system. Three levels of government—Commonwealth, state/territory and local—deliver the Australian health care system that is broadly divided into institutional and non institutional services. Institutional health services include public and private acute and psychiatric hospitals and residential aged care facilities. Non institutional services comprise medical services under Medicare, pharmaceuticals subsidised by the Pharmaceutical Benefits Scheme (PBS), and community health services and assistance.

The Commonwealth is responsible for GPs through the Medicare scheme and Medical Benefits Scheme, the PBS, the health of veterans and war widows, residential aged care and private health insurance. States and territories are responsible for public hospitals, public health services, community and mental health, home and community care and health promotion. Local governments deliver diverse levels and types of health related activities and services, usually relevant to and driven by local needs. Examples include sponsorship of health promotion and illness prevention activities; women's and men's health centres; ownership and support of residential aged care facilities; and youth support programs. And it is this breaking up of fiscal responsibility which works against ensuring that patient management between institutions and the community and between hospitals and GPs is continuous and effective.

The Medicare scheme is a universal health insurance system that covers all people resident in Australia. The Medicare principles are:

- *Choice of services:* Eligible persons must be given the choice to receive public hospital services free of charge as public patients.
- *Universality of services:* Access to public hospital services is to be on the basis of clinical need. An eligible person's priority for services will not be determined by whether or not they have health insurance, their financial status, place of residence, etc.
- *Equity in service provision:* To the maximum practicable extent, a state will ensure the provision of public hospital services equitably to all eligible persons, regardless of their geographical location. This principle does not require a local hospital to be equipped to provide each person with every hospital service they may need. In rural and remote areas, a state should ensure provision of reasonable public access to a basic range of hospital services, which are in accord with clinical practices.

Health care is the modern day equivalent of ancient Rome's Colosseum. It is the centre stage where gladiatorial battles are waged over funding, access and quality of care. The winners in the past have been politicians and/or major medical groups (Sax 1984). In the 1990s the economic rationalist's paradigm dominated the organisation, delivery and evaluation of health care. Evidence of such economic rationalists' policies can be observed through governments' rationing of health services, closure of hospitals, deregulation and restructuring of services and providers, and implementation of market based funding systems. Health care delivery began to look like a human production line, the primary function of which was the provision of diagnostic and therapeutic medical services (Palmer & Freeman 1991). It was the implementation of such policies that drew the critique that health had shifted to a market place mentality, trading health as a commodity.

PRESSURES ON THE HEALTH CARE SYSTEM

It is certainly the case that in health care systems in many countries in the world policy makers, consumers, professionals and politicians are being challenged. There is also evidence that the context in which care is delivered and the ideological basis upon which it has been developed are changing (Leeder 1999). A major challenge facing consumers and providers of health care services through the increased demand for services is how appropriately to meet such demands. In addition to the cost of increasing use of technology and changing community expectations, the changing demographic and social trends will also create an increasing burden on health and welfare systems. Our population is living longer, there is increasing urbanisation, changing family structures and we are a more multi-cultural society with increasing intergenerational gaps between the rich and poor (AIHW 1998b).

More educated and informed consumers already expect safer and more personalised health care services although it could be claimed that this should be routine in any health care system. The differences between those babies born before and during the Second World War, those born immediately after ('baby boomers') and the 'x-generation' will become more apparent. With the last two groups expecting greater choice, exploring and using complementary therapies, desiring health services to be located more conveniently and increasingly evaluating health care services through information technology such as the internet, consumer expectation will rise (AHMAC 1996).

New diseases, changing patterns of existing disease and environmental threats also deserve attention in terms of their impact on health care. These include infectious diseases such as tuberculosis and hepatitis and the problems posed by emerging antibiotic resistance as well as the problems associated with ageing, including neurodementias and musculoskeletal disorders, cancers, diabetes, drug and alcohol dependence and mental illness (AHMAC 1996).

Meanwhile technological advances, particularly in minimally invasive surgery, diagnostic and therapeutic interventions, genetic engineering and cybernetics are driving a revolution in the clinical care of patients. These factors require innovative approaches to service delivery, innovations that are consistent with health gain, providing higher levels of service and responsiveness. Along with such changes the necessity arises for specialist nurses, doctors, therapists, allied health practitioners and pharmacists all requiring education, not to mention research dollars.

Over the next decade predictions are that acute hospitals will be smaller, much smaller, with high dependency units and nearly four out of five medical/surgical beds will be monitored. The three 'big Cs' will continue to predominate—cancer, cardiac and casualty (trauma). Telemedicine will be routine in country areas, as will virtual reality robotics based surgery, physically separating the doctor from the patient. Gene therapy will be the antibiotic of the twenty-first century, most nursing will be provided in the home and nursing homes will more closely resemble the acute care facilities of today (Picone 1998).

The performance of the Australian health care system

What we are doing well

In 1991, Australia's expenditure on health care was 8.4% of GDP, the average for member countries of the Organisation for Economic Co-operation and Development (OECD). In comparison, the United States spends 14.0%, Canada spends 9.6% and the United Kingdom 6.9% (AIHW 1999). We have good life expectancy rates (although this is not so in our indigenous population) and people with acute illnesses generally receive prompt and high quality health care services. Ambulance response times are short, we have good trauma management and management of acute chest pain (NSW Department of Health 1998). Deaths due to coronary heart disease (CHD), stroke and asthma have been declining in NSW while smoking levels have dropped by around one-third since 1977 (NSW Department of Health 1998). But young people are still taking up smoking in large numbers, which highlights the need for new preventive health strategies.

Australian hospitals have certainly improved efficiency over the period 1993–94 to 1996–97, during which time the average length of stay for public hospitals fell by 11.5% from 6.1 to 5.4 days. However, the trend of shortening length of stay has done little to curtail soaring health care costs since average per capita costs continue to increase despite the decreasing bed days. This is because hospital stay is now far more expensive and patient throughput has not been, nor can it reasonably be, capped because of increased demand. Of course, this does not preclude debates about what we are now able to afford as a population and who should have priority to services. After all, such conversations are held, if ever, behind closed doors by those with vested interests. Public debate in this area might open a whole new definition of efficiency in terms of individual lives, not just length of stay. This would move the balance so that effectiveness was viewed as equally important as efficiency.

The majority of Australians support the principle of universal access to health care as enshrined in the Medicare arrangements since this guarantees them treatment services when needed. If we can believe the current debate conducted in the media, including letters and comments by consumers, most people feel deeply concerned about any proposal to dismantle Medicare, which would, in their view, be the beginning of a highly undesirable 'American style' health care system.

Areas where we could improve

But there are many areas in which we have not done so well. There remain significant differences in health outcomes for Aboriginal and Torres Strait Islander people. This is particularly evident in life expectancy and infant mortality rates. The health of people living in rural and remote Australia is also worse than those living in metropolitan areas (AIHW 1998a). Such health outcomes are not acceptable in a country that prides itself on an equitable health care system.

It is also a fact that the health system does not appropriately manage to fund the health needs of people with complex and chronic conditions such as those with respiratory diseases, cardiovascular diseases, cancer, mental disorders, and older persons with complex multi-systems disorders. Some of this occurs because of the fragmentation of services across GPs, acute and community care. The training of health care professionals, funding arrangements and the structure of the health care system have resulted in the system focusing on illness in hospitals rather than the quality of life of the general population and the provision of community delivered services.

Inefficiencies in the system such as duplication, unnecessary servicing, poorly planned services and fragmentation are certainly costly, not only to the system but also for the person. For example, the same diagnostic tests are repeated by the GP, a specialist and a hospital with people frequently ending up in hospital due to failed community support services. Some individuals repeatedly present for care in acute services such as hospital emergency departments, receiving treatment in acute care services because care is not coordinated with the community or the GP. This occurs in many, but not all, cases. Included in these phenomena are people with heart failure, respiratory disorders, vascular disease, drug and alcohol dependence, mental and developmental disorders and people with inadequate social and housing support. Coordinating such care requires the various government departments to acknowledge that health determinants are much wider than whether there is a hospital in the area. They include adequate housing, nutrition, education and employment.

Recent Australian research demonstrates that there is considerable room for improvement in the way we manage our acute hospital resources (Formby et al. 1991; Hathaway, Picone & Aisbett 1996; Picone, Ferguson & Hathaway 1993). Palmer and Freeman (1991) have indicated that a significant portion of hospital bed days is either unnecessary or inappropriate. Patients are being admitted or maintained in acute health care facilities for services or care that could be provided more efficiently in other health care settings, such as ambu-latory services or the home. There are also cost variations across similar groups of patients for the amount and complexity of care, patterns of care and length of stay (Hindle 1994). Added to this, most Australian health services still do not possess information technology systems to decide which treatments are effective, what clinical indi-cators are appropriate to measure the outcomes of health care interventions, and what outcomes we should expect from our health care interventions. This lack of adequate information technology is a major barrier when it comes to identifying what works and what doesn't, what is efficiently managed and what is inefficient.

Noticeably and notably the community is rarely engaged in dis-cussion or debate about the structure, funding and delivery of health care services yet they are the ones for whom the system should be working. Funders, providers, policy makers and governments make most of the decisions about funding and delivery of services, although there are pockets of consumer driven debate. Mainly, however, the government has failed to engage the community in these issues because health is primarily seen as political rather than welfare discourse.

HEALTH CARE AS A MARKET PLACE

Competition has been seen by many of the decision makers as the panacea for the problems in the Australian health care system thus introducing market place methodologies into health. Government, policy makers, private sector providers and many commentators believe that the efficiency of the health care sector could be signifi-cantly improved by increasing competition, thereby reducing the overall cost structure of health care through reducing inefficiencies such as long waiting lists (Refshauge 1995).

The public health care system is in many respects the opposite of a market place however, since the providers such as doctors and nurses operate monopolies (although it must be acknowledged that monop-olies also exist in large business corporations). Products are not easily defined and very few can be placed into the market place as a commodity of choice. Consumers are rarely able to exercise the choice experienced in the purchase of other commodities, sometimes due to ignorance and a sense of powerlessness, but sometimes due to cost. Finally, generally the community views the health service not as a commodity but as a highly significant public good, a fundamental social right. Further, the community expects government to intervene by both providing and regulating health services and protecting them from prevalent market forces such as private health corporations.

Given the lack of inherent market forces within health, competition has to be artificially constructed. This construction has been primarily achieved by the deliberative introduction of structural changes which mimic the market place. Such changes have included casemix payment systems, purchaser/provider arrangements, and deregulation of major providers and managed care. The most contentious method, casemix, is further explored below.

Casemix: A case study in market and competition policy

Casemix refers to the numbers of each type of patient category treated within a health care setting. Casemix in the Australian acute hospital sector is described using the ANDRG (Australian National Diagnosis Related Group) classification system (3M and MHI Systems 1993). Each ANDRG represents a class of patients with similar clinical conditions (clinical coherence) requiring similar resource usage (KPMG 1994).

The decision to pursue the development of casemix classification and payment systems in Australia was given impetus in the context of the 1988 Medicare Agreements. Since 1988 casemix systems, particularly classification and payment methods, have steadily evolved and developed both at national and state levels.

The implementation of casemix funding formulae in Victoria and South Australia was intended to improve allocative efficiency (utilisation patterns of in-patient services) and technical efficiency (practice patterns of clinicians and management of health facilities). Casemix funding was also expected to address issues relating to increasing costs and utilisation of health care services and cost variations across hospitals.

In Victoria the market place approach was made quite explicit as casemix funding was introduced across the health system. As the Secretary of the Department of Health and Community Services claimed shortly after the introduction of casemix funding in Victoria in July 1993: 'Within a short time the economics of the operations of public hospitals, individually and as a system, will become indistinguishable from Target, Safeway, General Motors Holden or McDonald's' (Paterson 1993).

Whether this is so or not, clinicians have certainly had considerable time and opportunity to debate and evaluate the many complex issues relating to casemix development in this country. Opinions remain polarised as to the benefits or otherwise of casemix payment systems and, interestingly, after nearly a decade of casemix development and implementation clinicians still view casemix with great suspicion. Perhaps this is because of its apparent goal to reduce costs. While casemix information as a classification system is effective in describing the work of hospitals, when it is used as a payment system clinicians believe casemix is detrimental to patient care (McCaughan & Picone 1997). Thus while some economists, academics, bureaucrats, politicians and hospital administrators present casemix as the panacea for improved hospital efficiency, for many clinicians casemix has become a populist apocalyptic metaphor for everything that is wrong with the health care system.

This is not to deny the usefulness of casemix as a tool for costing services. Using casemix data, it has been possible in a number of national and state costing studies to model total costs against casemix, producing a set of 'cost weights' (DHSH 1995). Cost weights are ratios of costs accrued by patients in one diagnosis related group to the average over all diagnosis related groups. Cost weights relate to the entire cost of a patient length of stay. Up until 1999 cost data have been restricted to the payment of patients treated in Victorian and South Australian hospitals only.

The difficulty in gaining an accurate picture of the strengths and weaknesses of casemix in action, apart from the problems reported by patients and clinicians, is a major barrier to further development of such a system nationally. The then Auditor-General of Victoria, in a thorough review of the Victorian casemix system (Baragwanath 1998), found a number of positive and negative features of the casemix payment system. It was found to be superior to previous funding systems in terms of efficiency gains, cost savings, improved access, and increased patient throughput. However, casemix payment failed to measure quality or patient outcomes, protect vulnerable patient groups at risk (chronically ill, elderly), or ensure continuity of care (Baragwanath 1998).

These findings are consistent with the findings of John Thompson (1988). Thompson commented in relation to post casemix implementation evaluation in North America that:

> As we go through this list of happenings in hospital care since April 1983 we will see that it is extremely difficult to determine whether they were caused by the DRG payment system (which some have characterised as a hospital acquired disease), whether they simply followed it, or whether they happened to occur at the same time that DRG payments were being implemented (Thompson 1988, p. 36).

One of the major problems with casemix is that it is not possible to assess the intended and unintended sequelae of casemix formulae. The reason for this is that the effects of casemix based funding formulae cannot be separated from the effects of the introduction of new technologies, changes in clinical practice and real funding reductions associated with increased demand. Thus, while casemix as a classification system contributes significantly to the description of workload of hospitals, it remains inadequate as a payment system and perhaps even counter-productive to patient care until severity, quality of care and patient outcomes (effectiveness) are included in the equations. A robust methodology is required linking casemix information to health outcomes, enhancing our ability to provide effective, appropriate, and cost effective clinical care to the Australian community (McCaughan & Picone 1997).

The argument against the health market place paradigm

Stockigt (1996) argues that current reforms to health funding and structures that are based on market and competition principles, including casemix funding, threaten the future of Australian public hospitals. Stockigt contends that policy makers and bureaucrats have capriciously adopted principles, structures and processes that essentially belong in production industries. The deliberative introduction of commercial or free market principles to complex human service industries such as health is fundamentally flawed, as both an economic and a social paradigm, the reason being health care by its very objectives and processes will always exhibit idiosyncratic behaviour in the market place. Health care is far more complex than a production line.

WHERE TO FOR THE AUSTRALIAN HEALTH CARE SYSTEM?

There are some immutable issues facing the Australian health care system. The pressures and demands of changing demographics and health technology will continue to place an increasing demand for health care services. If this demand is not managed, there will be major increases in health outlays relative to other human service agencies, outlays which will become so significant that society will not be able to fund them.

The old cost cutting methods of slashing through departments and functions do not necessarily provide longer term strategic solutions, quality patient care or satisfied clinical staff. Competition policy or the management of health as a market place, introduced through casemix, funder–provider arrangements and managed care, have had mixed outcomes and are not currently or likely to improve the effectiveness or efficiency of the Australian health care system.

For such a complex system in a changing society, a single solution is not only impossible, it may be inappropriate, although many decision makers prefer such near sighted solutions. In this case there is no magic bullet or it would have been found. There are many solutions however, some of which have not gained an airing and will never be aired because they cut across vested interests. One has only to look back at the unfolding of our present system and to note the comments made by Sax in 1984 regarding the two players who have had the most influence on our present system: politicians and doctors (medical practitioners). Politicians have driven the system forward because of entrenched ideology and doctors because of their need to remain independent from government interference. It appears that there are some definite features required to reform the health care system. Many of these ideas arose from a meeting convened in October 1995 by the Australian Health Ministers Advisory Council (AHMAC). This meeting of clinicians, consumers, policy makers, opinion leaders and commentators commissioned a paper on the preferred future of the Australian health care system (AHMAC 1996). The major recommendations from this paper are precised below.

- Care delivery systems—Australia's health system in 2010 should:
  - work affirmatively with and resource Aboriginal and Torres Strait Islander people to ensure their health years of life match those of non-indigenous people
  - provide equitable health care to all Australians according to need
  - move progressively towards a system where interventions depend upon evidence of cost effective benefit for prevention, care, cure, or palliation
  - offer a simple consumer friendly process to obtain comprehensive coordinated care
  - provide a primary health care-led system of integrated services which are closer to peoples homes and communities, in both urban and rural settings, and those in regional centres of excellence
  - integrate care by ensuring linkages between care systems, which reflect how the patient/client moves through the health care system rather than institutional, bureaucratic or professional

organisation—integrated care can be achieved through a variety of coordinated care service delivery models.

- Health practices that are effective—Australia's health system in 2010 should ensure that:
    - clinical guidelines are developed to help clinicians deliver the most appropriate and safe treatment to people
    - consumers are informed so that they can make informed decisions about treatment methods of independent evaluation and publication of comprehensive performance indicators
    - better information systems, such as integrated records and performance measures are developed—these systems would permit exchange of information between providers and improve care coordination.

- Financing and structure—Australia's health system in 2010 should:
    - incorporate payment arrangements which promote continuity of care
    - incorporate incentives for efficient provision of care and for rationalisation of services
    - be a coherent integrated system, eliminating conflicting policy directions from different/competing levels of government
    - provide incentives for appropriate coordinated care
    - possibly provide capitation payments for purchasing all the health care needs of an individual—these payments should provide incentives for encouraging a focus on prevention and more cost-effective services.

CONCLUSION

If implemented, these reforms will take many years to activate. Meanwhile there is no doubt that certain areas, namely rural and regional Australia, the health of indigenous people, private health insurance, and the anti-competitive practice of medical specialties require immediate attention by federal and state governments. But any progress of reform requires collaboration by the Commonwealth and states, the nursing and medical profession and most especially the Australian community. What is most evident is the need to stop the reform talk fest, stop piecemeal attempts at reforms based on market and competition policy and get on with the job of reshaping our health care system to meet the challenges. It is now time for action.

REFERENCES

Australian Health Ministers Advisory Council (AHMAC) (1996) *Australia's Health System in 2010*, Kilmore: Australian Health Ministers Advisory Council.

Australian Institute of Health and Welfare (AIHW) (1998a) *The Sixth Biennial Report of the Australian Institute of Health and Welfare: Australia's Health*, Canberra: AIHW.

AIHW (1998b) *Australia's Health 1998*, Canberra: AIHW.

AIHW (1999) *Health Expenditure Bulletin No. 15: Australia's Health Services Expenditure to 1997–98*, Health and Welfare Expenditure Series, Canberra: AIHW.

Baragwanath, C. (1998) *Special Report No. 56: Acute Health Services Under Casemix: A Case of Mixed Priorities*, Melbourne: Victorian Auditor-General's Office.

Department of Human Services and Health (DHSH) (1995) *Report on the Development of AN-DRG Version 3 Cost Weights and Supplementary Tables*, Canberra: DHSH.

Duckett, S. (1999) 'Policy challenges for the Australian health care system', *Australian Health Review*, vol. 22, no. 2, pp. 130–47.

Formby, D.J., McMullin, N.D., Danagher, K. and Oldham, D.R.A. (1991) 'The appropriateness evaluation protocol: Application in an Australian children's hospital', *Australian Clinical Review*, vol. 4, no. 11, pp. 123–31.

Hathaway, V., Picone, D. and Aisbett, C. (1996) *Version 3 AN-DRG Nursing Costing Study*, Sydney: Sydney Metropolitan Teaching Hospitals Nursing Consortium.

Healthcover (1999) 'Minister to establish health council to review NSW health care system', Press Release: Office of the Minister for Health, Sydney: Office of the NSW Minister for Health.

Hindle, D. (1994) *Product Costing: The Costing of Health Care Services*, Canberra: National Casemix Education Series.

Independent Pricing and Regulatory Tribunal of NSW (IPART) (1998) *Report to the NSW Treasurer and the Minister for Health: A Review of NSW Health*, Sydney: IPART.

KPMG (1994) *National Costing Study: Production of Cost Weights for AN-DRGs Version 2: A Report for the Commonwealth Department of Health and Human Services*, Canberra: KPMG Peat Marwick.

Leeder, S. (1999) *Healthy Medicine*, Sydney: Allen & Unwin.

McCaughan, B. and Picone, D. (1997) 'Casemix—not guilty', *Medical Journal of Australia*, vol. 167, no. 18, pp. 182–3.

NSW Department of Health (1998) *Health NSW 1998: The Chief Health Officer's Report on the Health of the People of New South Wales*, Sydney: NSW Department of Health.

Office of the Minister for Health (NSW) (1999) 'Media release 1: Minister to establish health council to review NSW health care system'.

Palmer, G. and Freeman, J. (1991) *Using DRGs for International Comparisons: DRGs Their Design and Development*, Ann Arbor: Health Administration Press.

Paterson, J. (1993) 'Beyond Case Payments: A New Paradigm for Australian Health and Welfare', in Economic Planning and Advisory Council, *Investing in Health: A Challenging Future*, Canberra: AGPS.

Picone, D. (1998) *Nursing in the Nanosecond Nineties and Beyond*, Annual Cardiac Nurses Conference, Coogee, NSW: Cardiac Nurses Association.

Picone, D., Ferguson, L. and Hathaway, V. (1993) *NSW Nursing Costing Study*, Sydney: Sydney Metropolitan Teaching Hospitals Nursing Consortium.

Refshauge, A. (1995) *Competition and Health Care*, Sydney: Lloyd Ross Forum.

Sax, S. (1984) *A Strife of Interests: Politics and Policies in Australian Health Services*, Sydney: Allen & Unwin.

Stockigt, J. (1996) 'Review: The commercialisation of public teaching hospitals is a fundamental error', *Medical Journal of Australia*, vol. 165, no. 9, pp. 482–4.

Thompson, J. (1988) 'DRG prepayment: Its purpose and performance', *Academic Medicine*, vol. 64, p. 35.

3M and MHI Systems (1993) *Australian National Diagnosis Related Groups Definitions Manual*, Sydney: Commonwealth Department of Human Services and Health.

COMMENTARY—CHAPTER 10

Kim Walker

A decided tension infuses current debates over how best to conceive Australia's health care system in these late capitalist, post-industrial, perhaps post-modern times. Is it an industry? A business? A market place? A social service mandated as a public right? These alternatives (among others) generate the tension just alluded to. It seems to me, however, with most of the western world firmly in thrall to economically rationalist fiscal policies—a phenomenon which some critical commentators have cleverly labelled 'market fundamentalism'—it is increasingly difficult to imagine how we might construct health as anything other than a market place.

Debbie Picone's chapter provides a largely descriptive account of a so-called 'health system' undeniably suffering and scarred from the effects of an all but global regime of truth. While she astutely points out the 'troubled and often anxious rhetoric that has continued almost unabated in relation to our health system', in narrating the state of 'health' in Australia, the rhetoric of crisis, collapse and chaos pervades her work as well. This suggests such rhetoric itself creates a particular reality that is neither 'actual' nor simply fabrication; the 'truth' probably lies somewhere messily in between.

Picone situates herself as a 'clinician, clinician manager and senior health executive' which indicates for me that collusion with such rhetoric is difficult, if not impossible to avoid. After all, as a senior health executive the author's need to conform with economically rationalist agendas and toe the line with market and competition driven policies must be all but an imperative on a daily basis. This may in part help us understand why we can talk of a 'crisis' that has a life of some two decades or more. Any suggestion that health is experiencing anything other than a 'crisis' is to disavow its authenticity and in so doing, health executives run the risk of having too few other arguments to beat-up those responsible for better funding and organising the 'system'.

In situating myself in relation to this critical commentary, I suggest the difference between myself and the author is that while much of my life has been as a clinician also, in latter years I have had the arguable luxury of standing somewhat outside of the hurly-burly of life in the delivery of health care and now sustain a vicarious, but nonetheless informed, relationship with this system.

For me then, a crisis that continues unabated for 20 years is not a 'crisis' but something much more sinister altogether. My metaphor of choice is that health can be thought of as inflicted with a malignancy both occult and overt at the same moment. Malignancies sometimes present as crises but in reality they effect their damage much more insidiously and much more deeply than a crisis often implies; they are also notoriously difficult to treat.

Perhaps the most telling moment in Picone's narrative comes about half-way through her chapter when she notes how little public debate and engagement in the funding and delivery of health care services has taken place. Those who have most to gain (and lose) from a market driven health care system have been systematically denied the privilege of input into that very system.

More disturbing still however, is her comment in relation to the soaring costs of health care—despite reductions in length of hospital stay—that increased demand of ever more expensive services continues to push costs through the ceiling. Picone tells us 'while this [situation] does not preclude debates about what we are now able to afford as a population and who should have priority to services . . . such conversations are held, if ever, behind closed doors by those with vested interests'.

This highlights a health care system, be it market place like or not, that is in the hands of many who have much to lose should we convert to a system driven by (rather than simply genuflecting toward) principles of equity of access, underpinned by the mobilisation of social capital, informed by an ethic of care and social justice, and which is attuned to effectiveness of outcomes not simply efficiencies of systems.

I ask: how did our health care system come to be colonised

by market forces, when in Picone's analysis it is neither, nor ought it to be conceived, as a market place in the first place? Whose interests have been served and whose needs met in this development? Health is not a simple commodity like a widget; in fact it is not a commodity at all. Health is a complex and little understood existential of humankind. This chapter makes excruciatingly clear at this time that through the very technologies we have invented and appropriated as humans to achieve our enlightenment, we have clung rather tenaciously, if not foolishly, to regimes of thought about health and illness that are deeply Cartesian—and therefore mechanistic, reductive and ultimately simplistic.

Picone feels compelled to recognise at the outset of her chapter that she 'describes a biomedical model of health . . . a model that focuses on an illness system, rather than a health system'. Such an admission for me explains, at least partially, why the economic fundamentalists will have their market place of health; their doctrines and dogma too, rest on essentially Cartesian and positivist foundations of the order of things. This said, we all will likely live to see the 'crisis' in health re-invent itself despite the reforms outlined in the closing pages of this chapter because such reforms issue from a world that bears little resemblance to the one we already inhabit and, sadly, with which too many of us are in deep complicity. Money makes the world go around, or so we have been seduced to believe; perhaps when we are able to recognise the paucity, not to mention the stupidity, of such a metaphor, we might have a health care system that is not a travesty of itself.

11 Always in the red

Kerry Russell

INTRODUCTION

Nursing services are essential for a hospital to achieve its objectives and outcome targets. Nursing provides a 24 hour clinical service and it is for this reason that this service usually accounts for the largest single component of a hospital's salaries and wages budget.

While nursing work is relatively invisible to many in health care services, it is far from invisible when translated into a hospital budget. Nurses are not in a position to raise revenue from their services and nursing is subsequently always in the red, showing up on the deficit side of the budget. In contrast, doctors are on the income side (in the black) since they are seen as bringing the goods (patients) into the hospital. This makes nursing an ideal target for cost reduction and constraint in a system constantly struggling for sufficient resources.

Nurse managers require high level skills to organise, plan and deliver health services that are top quality, cost effective and efficient. The old methods of resource management based on rebound responses do not provide longer term strategic solutions to resource management, quality patient care or staff satisfaction.

This chapter details a business planning model for the management of nursing resources and a rostering model, both of which allow nurses to have greater control of the management and use of health resources and the capacity to adjust staffing according to the level of activity.

BUSINESS PLANNING MODEL FOR THE MANAGEMENT OF NURSING RESOURCES

A major challenge facing health service providers is how to respond to changes in health care delivery associated with the increase in demand for services created by the growth and ageing of the population, changing community expectations and a technology driven revolution in the clinical management of patients. These factors, coupled with changes to funding mechanisms, require innovative approaches to service delivery. We need to ensure such innovations are commensurate with health gain, provide higher levels of service and responsiveness, and are contestable in the health market. Health care clinicians and managers are accountable for this increasingly complex matrix of health care delivery, management and organisation.

The business planning model has been developed by Debbie Picone and Kerry Russell over a number of years and it has been used and remodelled when consulting with hospitals across Australia. It is a step by step method of examining nursing resource requirements, taking into account a range of qualitative and quantitative data that impact on service delivery. The model relates to finances, staffing and broader issues such as ward design. It uses a systematic approach to examining the current situation and determining future staffing requirements given the available resources. It constructs a framework for the effective use of nursing resources within the prevailing economic paradigm that recognises the complex tapestry of care provided by nurses in acute care facilities.

The aim of the model is to improve efficiency and effectiveness. It is based on consultation with key stakeholders and industrial associations, and it must fit with the long term goals and objectives of the organisation.

There are four interrelated stages of the business planning model:

1. review of whole of health facility
2. review of individual units
3. alignment of staffing resources to clinical service requirements
4. compilation of summary staffing plan.

The model is based on an algorithm, which reflects and interacts with the reality of contemporary clinical care, health service management and nursing service organisation. The methodology is detailed in Table 11.1.

Table 11.1   Stages of the business planning model for the management of nursing resources

Stage	Activity
1. Review whole of health facility	• Examine role and function of health facility including organisation structure • Examine key issues and pressures • Review budget issues • Review service activity, including throughput data • Review fixed nursing costs — Average annual salary — Staffing profile — Casual staff utilisation • Examine nursing organisation structure and delegations for resource management Examine casemix data including top 15 ANDRGs
2. Review individual units (which represent a nursing cost centre)	• Develop a clinical profile • Develop a staffing profile • Monitor activity levels • Ascertain top 10 ANDRGs by relative frequency • Review average nursing intensity • Ascertain issues that affect workload • Ascertain nursing hours per patient day • Create an annual unit bed management plan
3. Align staffing resources to clinical service requirements	In line with available resources, develop a master unit plan for each unit recommending: • Productive full time equivalent (FTE) requirements • Additional day off (ADO) and leave relief FTE requirements • Total FTE requirements
4. Compile summary staffing plan	• Detail findings • Develop staffing and salaries/wages plan for whole of nursing service • Monitor actual staff utilisation against plan

Step 1: Review of whole of health facility

This step involves examining the role and function of the health facility, focusing on key issues and pressures, and budgetary issues. This may include clinical service changes—for example, the introduction of cardiac surgery or a decrease in the number of available beds—as well as any budget overrun that may need to be carried forward.

Next, service activity is reviewed. This includes throughput data, which should be examined for the past three years as well as the projected current year. Activity data over a three year period will identify trends and provide a strategic view of what is happening within the organisation in terms of its activity. This information can be compared with staffing trends for the same period. An example of the information required is detailed in Appendix 11.1.

Fixed nursing costs are also reviewed and staffing trends analysed, including average annual salary, staffing profile and casual staff utilisation. Benchmarking with similar facilities can be undertaken to determine whether these costs are appropriate. Information required for the analysis of staffing trends is detailed in Appendix 11.2.

The nursing organisation structure and delegations is then examined for resource management. Opportunities for sharing resources across a number of health facilities should be considered where appropriate.

Finally, casemix data should be examined, including top 15 ANDRGs by relative volume. This can provide valuable information in terms of describing clinical workload and determining average nursing intensity on an individual unit basis.

Step 2: Review of individual units

Individual units are reviewed through the development of a clinical and staffing profile and master unit plan (Appendixes 11.3 and 11.4).

A clinical profile for each unit and department is developed and used to determine required staffing levels. The profile includes a description of the main clinical casemix, activity levels, staff skillmix and any particular characteristics of the unit that affects workload. The information required differs depending on the nature of the unit. However, in general, for 24 hour clinical units the following information is collected:

- *Activity levels* for the previous year including total bed days, separations, average occupancy and average length of stay. Activity from other areas may include outpatient or day-only occasions of service, emergency department attendances, emergency department admission rate and triage categories, and total operations performed. Table 11.2 provides definitions for a range of factors that affect hospital activity levels.

- *Staffing details* including the current year staffing level (for which funding is available), annual leave and sick leave relief provision, actual full time equivalent (FTE) used in the previous year, actual FTE used in the year to date, casual staff utilised (agency and casual pool), and funded and actual nursing hours per patient day. Staffing details also relate to skillmix and any particular staffing characteristics that affect the workload (e.g. staff who act as preceptors for undergraduate nursing students).
- *Clinical details* describing the main clinical casemix of the unit.
- *Workload characteristics* describing any particular features of the unit that affects workload and subsequent staffing requirements such as ward design and layout, number of surgical operating days per week and annual ward closures over the Christmas/New Year period. It also relates to support staff available to the unit, including secretarial, allied health and portering services.
- *Top 15 ANDRGs per unit by relative volume* describing the highest volume ANDRGs of each unit for the previous year and/or year to date, and assigning nursing intensity weights to each ANDRG.

Step 3: Alignment of staffing resources to clinical service requirements

This step is where all the information is analysed and recommendations on clinical service realignments are formulated. These assessments should be consistent with best contemporary clinical management practice in Australia. For example, it is necessary to examine what the implications will be (clinically and financially) of the proposed realignment to services and/or staffing resources.

As part of this stage, a master unit plan is developed for each unit/department. An example of a master unit plan and salaries and wages budget buildup is provided in Appendix 11.4. The master unit plan is built up on a shift by shift basis. It takes into account the shifts required on a seven day and Monday to Friday basis. From this, the total FTE required is determined. The plan should be accompanied by a corresponding salaries and wages budget based on an appropriate

Table 11.2 Definitions of factors that affect hospital activity levels

Number of beds	The number of available beds or treatment chairs (e.g. dialysis chairs) that are immediately available to be used for treatment of patients admitted into the unit; that is, it is resourced with services and staff and is located in a suitable place for care.
Total occupied bed days	The total number of bed days of all inpatients who were separated during the year, excluding leave days. A formal separation is a discharge, transfer or death of a patient. Details for same-day separations are also recorded as inpatient bed days where one inpatient bed day is counted for each same-day separation.
Average length of stay	The average length of stay for all inpatients (excluding same-day patients). All bed days accumulated by the patient at the time the patient separates should be counted.
Occupancy rate	The percentage of available beds that have been occupied over the year. The bed occupancy rate is a measure of intensity of the use of hospital resources by inpatients.
Occasions of service	An output measure of health care services provided to non-inpatients. An occasion of service is defined as any examination, consultation, treatment or other service provided to a patient in each functional unit of a health care establishment. Types of non-inpatient services include: • Individual services, where a single patient receives one or more non-inpatient service directly from a health care professional attached to a functional unit of a health care facility and a record is made of the occasion showing the nature of the service(s) provided. • Group services, where a group of non-inpatients receives health care service(s) directly from an employee of a functional unit of a health care facility and a record is made of the occasion showing the nature of the service(s) and the number of participants.
Episode of care	A phase of treatment during which the patient receives a particular type of care (e.g. acute rehabilitation). When that type of care is concluded, the episode of care is ended and the patient undergoes either a type change separation to a different type of care or a formal separation and leaves the hospital.

Table 11.2 continued

Emergency department presentations	The number of patients who arrive at to an emergency department of a hospital.
Percentage of admissions through emergency department	The proportion of all emergency department separations where the patient was admitted through the emergency department.
Triage scale	A process of scoring patients according to the urgency of assessment and treatment required. Patients are placed into one of five categories on the National Triage Scale according to the triageur's response to the question: 'This patient should wait no longer than . . .'.

Source: NSW Department of Health 1997

staff profile. The total FTE for each unit should take the following into account:

- Headcount required per shift, including seven day shiftworkers and Monday to Friday requirements
- Additional day off (ADO) relief requirements
- Annual leave relief requirements in accordance with the relevant award. In New South Wales, for example, this would be calculated on the following basis: seven day shiftworkers, 228 hours (six weeks) relief per FTE; non shiftworkers, 152 hours (four weeks). It may be appropriate to reduce the annual leave relief provision that is built into the unit FTE on the basis that not all employees accrue their full leave entitlement due to staff turnover. In addition, the leave liability which most hospitals constantly strive to reduce indicates that a significant number of nurses do not take their full leave entitlement. Where there is an annual closure of a unit it is suggested that annual leave relief either not be built into the FTE or be reduced, depending on the duration of the closure.
- Sick leave relief, where provision should be made for five days relief on the basis that not all sick leave needs to be replaced due to varying levels of activity and occupancy rates as well as the potential for redeployment from other units. It is suggested that funding (but not FTE) for sick leave relief be built into the unit budget and that the relief be provided through a casual pool of nurses employed by the facility. A further option for managing the provision of supplementary staff is discussed in the section entitled 'Unit managed staffing'.

- Funded nursing hours per patient day (NPPD), calculated on the productive FTE staffing level and average occupancy. It is suggested that the nursing unit manager and ward secretary (if part of the nursing budget) be excluded from the NPPD. Benchmarking between like units can be performed on the basis of NPPD and nursing intensity weights; however, it is important not to rely solely on NPPD but to consider the variations identified in the clinical profile.

Step 4: Compilation of summary staffing plan

The summary staffing plan consists of the individual unit staffing levels (productive/non productive), corresponding salaries and wages budget, NPPD and average occupancy. It provides a detailed account of the nursing salaries and wages budget against which actual staff utilisation can be monitored to ensure that actual staffing levels match the resources available (see Appendix 11.5).

UNIT MANAGED STAFFING: AN INNOVATIVE APPROACH TO ROSTERING

The unit managed staffing (UMS) model is an innovative model of staffing based, in part, on the unit based staffing model used at The Alfred Hospital, Melbourne (The Alfred Hospital 1998) and the Aberdeen annual hours model developed in Scotland (Allanach 1998, pp. 33–6). The UMS model will be introduced as a pilot project at Concord Repatriation General Hospital, a facility of the Central Sydney Area Health Service (CSAHS) and a teaching hospital of the University of Sydney, in line with the CSAHS's commitment to the recruitment and retention of nurses.

Issues relating to recruitment and retention of the nursing workforce have been identified in a multitude of reports. One of the most recent reports focusing on recruitment and retention is that produced by the NSW Ministerial Nursing Recruitment and Retention Taskforce (NSW Health 1996) which identifies issues such as the need for family-friendly, flexible work practices, more effective management of workload and staffing, improved work relationships, rewards and recognition, better communication and access to professional networks.

Nurses often perceive that they have a lack of control over staffing at the unit level. The ad hoc redeployment of nurses to other units to cover unplanned shortages is common, and there is an increasing use of agency staff, often unfamiliar with the hospital, unit and specialty. Similarly, nurses traditionally have had little or no control over unit activity. It is driven primarily by the activities of Medical Officers and is affected by school holidays, periods of leave and medical conferences. The UMS model was developed in an attempt to address these issues.

UMS is a means by which nurses can gain increased rostering flexibility and the capacity to adjust staffing levels on the basis of clinical activity. Subject to effective management, it is cost neutral and has the potential to promote a professional service, and enhance the retention of nurses through increased job satisfaction. UMS is particularly beneficial in areas that have significant peaks and troughs in activity.

Methodology

UMS is a method that allows nurses to accumulate credit or debit hours, also known as 'bank hours', which are taken or paid back at a time negotiated with the manager. It functions independently of the standard rostering practice, the basis of which remains the relevant nurses award. It needs to be emphasised that the methodology for the UMS model may be outside of the award under which nurses work and must therefore be subject to union and Health Department (or equivalent) negotiation and agreement prior to implementation.

It is anticipated that UMS will provide nurses with a higher level of job satisfaction through increased rostering flexibility, more control over staffing at the unit level and the ability to adjust staffing on the basis of clinical activity. It is also anticipated that higher levels of satisfaction will result in improved patient outcomes through increased continuity of care. Benefits will need to be identified through effective methods of evaluation.

Sample framework

The key elements of UMS are mutual agreement and negotiation. The project should be administered within a clearly defined set of guidelines. Factors that should be covered in these guidelines are given below.

Participation

Participation in UMS is on a voluntary basis and is available to full time and part time registered nurses, enrolled nurses and assistants in nursing.

Management of unplanned staffing shortages

This will be through either the standard rostering process or by negotiating with participants of UMS to either accumulate or pay back hours.

Accumulation of credit/debit hours

Accumulation of credit/debit hours is on the basis of the employee's standard hours of employment and there will be no access to additional ordinary hours of pay under these arrangements, unless or until the maximum accrued under the UMS arrangement is exceeded.

- Employees who participate in UMS may accumulate additional hours or take time off up to a limit of 30 hours. A limit of 30 hours has been established on the basis of it being a manageable level for both employee and employer.
- Nurses may accumulate credit/debit hours within the 30 hour limit spanning a period of 12 months from 1 July to 30 June each year. There is no benefit in restricting the period to less than 12 months. Any shorter period will only serve to reduce flexibility.
- Hours should be neutral upon resignation date. The administrator of UMS is responsible for ensuring that the employee is able to take credit hours owing to the employee prior to the termination date. Outstanding hours upon termination date will be paid out or deducted from the termination pay at the ordinary rate of pay.
- Hours will be neutral upon transfer of the employee to another clinical unit.
- Accumulation of credit/debit hours will be with the prior approval of the nurse manager of the unit (or person in charge).
  Hours owed to the unit will be paid back through an availability roster, an example of which is located in Appendix 11.6. This is a roster, posted in the unit, where nurses who owe hours can indicate times they are available to pay back those hours. There must be no coercion to pay back hours at times that do not suit employees.
- By virtue of placing themselves on the availability roster employees are not regarded as being on-call. Employees are not obliged to return to work if requested.
- The minimum credit/debit time for which hours may be accumulated is 30 minutes, with prior authorisation of the nurse manager or delegate.
- The model must not be a process to address poor time management skills. Should the workload require additional resources, 30 minutes is considered a reasonable timeframe.

- There will be no UMS activity on public holidays; that is, employees are not permitted to either debit or credit their hours on these days.

Calculation of credit/debit hours

As identified previously, UMS functions independently, but alongside the standard rostering and payroll system. The existing method for signing-off employees standard hours is maintained. That is, employees are signed off for the hours they are scheduled to work, including any overtime worked and leave taken.

Accumulation of hours under UMS is not considered leave (for debit hours) or overtime (for credit hours). An employee who under UMS continues to work following the completion of the shift, or leaves prior to the completion of the shift, will accumulate either credit or debit hours in their 'bank'. These UMS hours are not entered into the payroll system and pay is not affected.

Penalty rates will be paid for hours not worked under UMS. For example, if an employee is rostered to work eight hours on Sunday but left after five hours (UMS debit hours) the employee will be signed off for an eight hour shift and paid penalty rates for eight hours. The employee will subsequently owe hours to the unit. As penalty rates have been paid for hours not worked, hours owed to the unit will be calculated at the penalty rate equivalent. In the above scenario, under the NSW Nurses Public Hospital State Award, if the nurse left three hours early on Sunday, they would owe five hours, 25 minutes to the unit. Accordingly, penalty rates will not be paid when debit hours are paid back. Employees have already received penalty rate payment for the hours not worked.

Debit and credit hours will be adjusted to the penalty rate equivalent in accordance with the relevant award. That is, the penalty rate adjusted hours will be normalised both ways. The adjustment will ensure fairness to both employee and employer. For example, it will overcome any incentive to take time off on Saturday/Sunday when penalty rates are paid and pay back hours owed on weekdays. The reverse scenario would also be applicable. On this basis, there are no incentives or disincentives in regard to hours owed or hours owing.

As UMS does not involve payment it will ensure that employees are not disadvantaged in terms of penalty rate entitlements. For example, if employees take time off on a weekday for which there is no penalty rate payment, and pay back hours on a Sunday, they would clearly be disadvantaged. Adjustment of the hours to a penalty rate equivalent on both a debit and credit basis will overcome any inequities. An Hours Accumulation Chart is shown in Appendix 11.7.

Meal breaks when making up hours

If an employee works more than two hours following the completion of a shift, a 20 minute meal break will be given, and further 20 minutes for each subsequent four hours worked. This is also the case if an employee is recalled to pay hours back for a period exceeding four hours.

If an employee volunteers to pay back hours on a rostered day off, then normal meal breaks for that shift will apply.

Maintaining of records

The current payroll signing-off process for standard hours is maintained, and the nurse manager will maintain an accurate register of UMS hours on a cumulative basis. The UMS register will span a 12 month period and UMS participants will be advised of their UMS status on a monthly basis.

Participants will sign the register at the completion of each roster period. At the completion of each roster period a copy of the UMS register will become an adjunct to the master roster and maintained for the required period of time.

The UMS register will be subject to three monthly audits, the results of which will be documented.

Duration of the trial

It is suggested that sites that introduce a UMS model do so through a pilot project for a 12 month period. There thould be an initial review at the completion of six months.

Review mechanisms

The following are some of the mechanisms that could be used to determine the effectiveness of UMS:

- Clinical indicators, including fails, pressure areas and medication errors. The rates should be analysed and compared to the previous 12 month period.
- Staff satisfaction survey, before and after the implementation of UMS.

- Monitoring and reporting on sick leave rates, agency staff usage and staff turnover. The rates should be analysed and compared to the previous 12 month period.
- Three monthly audits to determine compliance with guidelines.
- Cost neutrality—agency staff and overtime expenditure should be examined before and after the implementation of UMS.

CONCLUSION

In conclusion, this chapter focused on nursing resources and covered two areas. It provided, first, an outline of one way in which nursing resources may be managed and, second, an innovative model to facilitate the adjustment of staffing on the basis of clinical activity.

Section 1 detailed a four step model which will facilitate the development of a nursing business plan, the aim of which is to facilitate the effective and efficient allocation and ongoing management of nursing resources based on clinical service needs. It is intended to replace the old 'across the board' cuts to nursing budgets which do not take into account the clinical workload of individual units. It is a cyclical process which should be undertaken routinely, on an annual basis. This plan also provides a framework to adjust staffing levels and budget allocation each time there are changes to a clinical service.

Section 2 described an innovative model of staffing, based on a credit/debit process of hours. It has been developed from the excellent models used in Victoria (unit based staffing) and Aberdeen (annual hours) in an attempt to increase continuity of care, facilitate staffing on the basis of clinical activity and importantly, to provide nurses with increased flexibility and control over their working lives.

REFERENCES

The Alfred Hospital (1998) *Site Visit*, Melbourne: unpublished records.

Allanach, H. (1998) 'Organising the workforce: Annual hours in nursing (management)', *Nursing Standard*, vol. 12, no. 24, March, pp. 33–6.

NSW Department of Health (1997) *NSW Public Hospitals Comparison Databook, 1996/97* Sydney: NSW Department of Health.

NSW Health (1996) *Nursing Branch Bulletin*, Nursing Recruitment and Retention Taskforce Report, August.

COMMENTARY—CHAPTER 11

Belinda Chaplin

In the early 1980s the 'hospital secretary' visited all the wards around June of each year to ask the Charge Sister to place an order for a non stock item, usually a piece of equipment, prior to the end of the year so that we would not have to give money back to the Health Commission. Those were the days when a patient after an appendectomy had a ten day stay in hospital, food was freshly prepared in the hospital kitchen and the wards had their own complement of housekeeping staff.

The first wave of reductions in hospital spending began in the early 1980s when the government commenced a round of hospital closures. The closures came quickly in New South Wales: Parramatta, Crown Street Women's, Eastern Suburbs and Marrickville Hospitals. At the same time new hospitals were opening out in the west of Sydney. Many of these years were spent fighting what seemed to be endless rounds of reductions in acute public hospital spending, particularly in Sydney's east.

The demands on the health dollar are not likely to decrease in the short term. Changing demographics such as population growth and ageing, rising community expectations, changes in clinical practice, expanding range of service provision, growth in non invasive surgical techniques, growing capacity to treat people and advancements in technology are all placing pressure on levels of health care expenditure.

Nurses are, with other health professionals, expected to closely examine the cost of health services. We have quickly become adept at budgeting and managing health resources. Kerry Russell gives two descriptive accounts of methods that enable nurses to influence the allocation of dollars in today's health care environment. The first is a new and more flexible approach to rostering practices. Nurses have rightly been critical of rigid rostering methods that are neither lifestyle- nor family-friendly. The unit managed staffing method gives control to the nurse clinicians and provides an opportunity for a more flexible approach to work hours. A hybrid of this method has been successful in a number of teaching hospitals and will no doubt be extended to other health care settings. The second is a method for developing a staffing plan within a hospital. At first appearance the method appears very complex, a reflection of the actual complexity of modern day health care provision. However, it provides a 'level playing field' for nurses to determine and argue for appropriate resource allocation in the face of almost endless competing priorities. The staffing method also ensures an equitable distribution of funding to various units and departments. Most importantly, the method will inform decisions regarding service levels if insufficient funds are available to provide health programs. Finally, the method in its current form would be greatly enhanced if informed by quality, effectiveness and staff satisfaction data.

Appendix 11.1

KEY ACTIVITY INDICATORS
(sample hospital)

Activity indicator	1996/97	1997/98	1998/99	Variation (%) 1996/97– 1998/99
Available beds	116	116	112	–3.45
Total separations	3 338	3 374	4 545	36.15
Same day	2 337	2 510	2 778	18.87
Not same day	1 001	1 224	1 767	76.52
Live births	104	110	98	–5.77
Bed days	30 631	31 000	35 441	15.70
ALOS (admission based)	9.18	8.3	7.8	–15.03
Bed occupancy rate	72%	73%	84%	16.67
Total operations performed	2 300	2 020	2 189	–4.83
Day only	1 201	1 210	1 280	6.58
Emergency dept attendances	3 001	2 090	2 431	–18.99
Emergency dept admission rate	6.00%	4.30%	4.70%	–21.67
Emergency dept triage scale				
Category 1	0.34%	0.08%	0.21%	–38.24
Category 2	0.83%	0.70%	0.80%	–3.61
Category 3	2.36%	2.10%	3.00%	27.12
Category 4	37.37%	28.30%	38.00%	1.69
Category 5	58.40%	68.80%	58.00%	–0.68
Annual trauma cases	20	25	18	–10
Major trauma	8	4	9	12.5
Minor trauma	12	21	9	–25

Appendix 11.2

ANALYSIS OF STAFFING TRENDS

Indicator	1996/97	1997/98	1998/99
Average number of total hospital staff (EFT)	240	239	237
Average number of nurses	102	100.6	99.7
Bed number	116	116	112
Nursing % of total hospital	**42.63%**	**42.14%**	**42.09%**

Note: 1998/99 data provided from July 1998 to November 1998. Extrapolated for full year.

Appendix 11.3

CLINICAL AND STAFFING PROFILE

Hospital   XXXX
Unit/Department Ward 1
Description   Acute Surgical and Medical Ward

Bed utilisation data 199697		Staffing details (current financial year)		Recommended NPPD and funded FTE
		Funded FTE 1997/98		**Funded FTE 1998/9**
Number of beds	18.0	Funded productive EFT 1997/98	13.70	13.81
Total occupied bed days	5 389	Sick leave relief	0.24	0.25
Annual separations	1 214	Annual leave relief	1.40	0.97
Average LOS (days)	4.60	Total funded EFT 1997/98	15.34	15.03
Occupancy rate	82%	Funded NPPD	4.29	4.34
ED attendances	n/a	**Actual FTE utilised**		
Average attendances/day	n/a	Productive FTE 1997/98	12.80	
Live births	n/a	Leave relief FTE used	1.30	
Non inpatient occasions of service	n/a	Agency FTE	2.00	
Number of theatres	n/a	Total FTE used YTD	16.10	
Total operations	n/a	Actual NPPD	4.33	
Average start time	n/a	Funded/actual variance FTE	0.76	
Average finish time	n/a	Funded/actual variance NPPD	0.04	
Theatre utilisation rate	n/a			

Notes: EFT = average number of total hospital staff; FTE = full time equivalent;
LOS = length of stay; NPPD = Nursing hours per patient per day; YTD = year to date

Clinical profile

> The ward provides services for the treatment and management of acute general and elective and emergency surgical patients. Surgical lists are scheduled each day from Monday to Friday.
>
> Types of surgery include primarily colo-rectal, ophthalmology, vascular and gynaecology. Medical admissions include a wide range of multi-systems problems as well as back pain and stroke.

Staffing profile

> This ward is staffed by a mix of registered nurses and enrolled nurses with a ratio of 4:1. There is a part time component of 28%. A ward clerk is rostered from Monday to Friday but is not a part of the nursing budget.
>
> The ward employs three new graduate nurses per year for whom the experienced nurses act as preceptors. Thirty-four per cent of registered nurses hold speciality qualifications relevant to the clinical casemix of the ward.

Workload characteristics

> The ward is consistently busy due to the acute nature of in-patients and the daily (Monday to Friday) operating lists.
>
> Medical admissions are often elderly, frail and dependent requiring the full range of nursing care.

Appendix 11.4

MASTER UNIT PLAN

Hospital	XXXX

Unit/Department	Ward 1
Description	Acute Surgical and Medical Ward
Bed number	18.0
Occupancy rate	82.0%

Seven day shift requirements

Monday to Friday	Morning	Evening	Night duty (8 hour shift)	Night duty (10 hour shift)
Headcount per shift (excl. NUM)	3.0	3.0	2.0	
Weekly EFT requirement	**3.00**	**3.00**	**2.00**	**0.00**

Saturday to Sunday	Morning	Evening	Night duty (8 hour shift)	Night duty (10 hour shift)
Headcount per shift (excl. NUM)	3.0	3.0	2.0	
Weekend multiplier	0.40	0.40	0.40	0.50
Weekly EFT requirement	**1.20**	**1.20**	**0.80**	**0.00**

Shift worker EFT requirements

Total Monday to Friday	8.00
Total Saturday to Sunday	3.20
Subtotal	**11.20**

Non-shift worker EFT requirement

Nursing Unit Manager	1.00
Other—Ward clerk/secretarial	1.00
Total	**2.00**

Total productive staff requirements	**13.20**

Note: Sick leave relief FTE is excluded from total roster requirements but the funding for sick leave relief is included in the total funded FTE.

Relief	
ADO relief	0.61
Subtotal	**13.81**
Holiday/sick leave relief	
Sick leave	0.25
Annual leave relief (note: reduced due to annual closure)	
a. Monday to Friday	0.04
b. Seven day shift workers	0.93
Subtotal annual/sick leave relief	**1.22**

Nursing hours per patient day	**4.34**
Total roster requirements	**14.78**
Total staff requirements	**15.03**

Notes: EFT = average number of total hospital staff; FTE = full time equivalent;
NUM = nursing unit manager

Appendix 11.5

1999/2000 BUDGET AND STAFFING PLAN (NURSING)
(Sample hospital)

Unit	\ 1999/2000 budget estimate \ Cost centre	Budget allocation $	Bed	Occ 1998/99	FTE 1999/00	A/L relief	Total rostered	S/L relief	Total funded FTE	Funded NPPD	M–F AM	M–F PM	M–F ND	Sat–Sun AM	Sat–Sun PM	Sat–Sun ND	Funded FTE 1998/99	S/L relief	A/L relief	Total funded FTE	1998/99 1999/00 variance (FTE)
Ward 1	30272	1 044 342	29	82%	22.63	1.22	23.85	0.42	24.27	4.71	8.00	5.00	3.00	6.00	5.00	3.00	22.63	0.42	1.24	24.29	-0.02
Ward 2	30292	966 703	9	80%	17.30	2.04	19.34	0.33	19.67	11.91	7.50	3.00	2.00	5.00	3.00	2.00	18.35	0.35	2.12	20.82	-1.15
Ward 3	30312	1 041 785	24	82%	21.37	2.48	23.85	0.40	24.25	5.34	8.00	5.00	3.00	5.00	4.00	2.00	21.37	0.40	2.48	24.25	0.00
Ward 4	30122	77 134	0	n/a	2.00	0.00	2.00	0.00	2.00	n/a	2.00	0.00	0.00	0.00	0.00	0.00	2.00	0.00	0.00	2.00	0.00
Endocrinology support	30121	58 666	0	n/a	1.00	0.00	1.00	0.00	1.00	n/a	1.00	0.00	0.00	0.00	0.00	0.00	1.00	0.00	0.00	1.00	0
Othopaedic support	30271	62 772	n/a	n/a	1.00	0.00	1.07	0.00	1.07	n/a	1.00	0.00	0.00	0.00	0.00	0.00	1.00	0.00	0.07	1.07	0
Diabetes education centre	30124	149 947	0	n/a	3.00	0.00	3.00	0.00	3.00	n/a	3.00	0.00	0.00	0.00	0.00	0.00	3.00	0.00	0.00	3.00	0
Burns support	30291	205 357	n/a	n/a	4.00	0.07	4.07	0.00	4.07	n/a	4.00	0.00	0.00	0.00	0.00	0.00	1.00	0.00	0.07	1.07	3
Trauma unit	30331	18 336	n/a	n/a	0.40	0.00	0.40	0.00	0.40	n/a	0.40	0.00	0.00	0.00	0.00	0.00	0.40	0.00	0.00	0.40	0
TOTAL		3 625 042	62		72.70	5.81	78.58	1.15	79.66		34.90	13.00	8.00	16.00	12.00	7.00	70.75	1.17	5.98	77.90	1.83

Notes: Agreed nursing hours per patient day (NPPD) excludes nursing unit manager and ward clerk

Daily staffing plan (AM shift) includes nursing unit manager and ward clerk

Total rostered FTE is the productive FTE and annual leave relief that is allocated to the ward. Sick leave relief FTE is not allocated to the ward

Total rostered FTE—Funding for sick relief is built into the ward budget to accommodate replacement casual staff

A/L = annual leave

S/L = sick leave

Appendix 11.6

UNIT MANAGED STAFFING
AVAILABILITY ROSTER
Roster period 1 January 2000 to 14 January 2000

Name	M	T	W	T	F	S	S	M	T	W	T	F	S	S
Smith, R.	AM 7–2		AM 7–1						PM 3–7					
Back, S.					PM 2–6								AM 9–4	
Cann, D.														
Hill, K.				PM 3–8				PM 3–7						
Higgs, G.														
Briggs, A.												AM 7–3		
South, Y.									AM 8–3	AM 8–3				
Pye, W.	PM 6–9													
West, P.														
Lye, B.													AM 7–3	

Appendix 11.7

UMS HOURS ACCUMULATION AND ADJUSTMENT CHART

Variation to hours (additional worked) (taken off)	Day shift (no penalties)	Evening shift 12.5%	Night shift 15%	Saturday 50%	Sunday 75%	Public holiday (no UMS activity)
1		7.5	9.0	30.0	45.0	Nil
Total time owed/owing	1 hr	1 hr, 8 mins	1 hr, 9 mins	1 hr, 30 mins	1 hr, 45 mins	
2		15.0	18.0	60.0	90.0	Nil
Total time owed/owing	2 hrs	2 hrs, 15 mins	2 hrs, 18 mins	3 hours	3 hrs, 30 mins	
3		22.5	27.0	90.0	135.0	Nil
Total time owed/owing	3 hrs	3 hrs, 23 mins	3 hrs, 27 mins	4 hrs, 30 mins	5 hrs, 25 mins	
4		30.0	36.0	120.0	180.0	Nil
Total time owed/owing	4 hrs	4 hrs, 30 mins	4 hrs, 36 mins	6 hrs	7 hrs	
5		37.5	45.0	150.0	225.0	Nil
Total time owed/owing	5 hrs	5 hrs, 38 mins	5 hrs, 45 mins	7 hrs, 5 mins	8 hrs, 45 mins	
6		45.0	54.0	180.0	270.0	Nil
Total time owed/owing	6 hrs	6 hrs, 45 mins	6 hrs, 54 mins	9 hrs	10 hrs, 30 mins	
7		52.5	63.0	210.0	315.0	Nil
Total time owed/owing	7 hrs	7 hrs, 53 mins	8 hrs, 3 mins	10 hrs, 30 mins	12 hrs, 15 mins	
8		60.0	72.0	240.0	360.0	Nil
Total time owed/owing	8 hrs	9 hrs	9 hrs, 12 mins	12 hrs	14 hrs	

Index

Aboriginal health 182, 183
abortion 150–1
Abortion Act 1966 (UK) 150
aged care 138–9
  cost versus quality 124–5
  legislation 124–5
  and nursing staff 124–5, 127, 128
  and pain 4
  rationalisation of 125–8
  residential 124, 126, 128–32,
    133–4, 138
Aged Care Act 124–5, 133, 138
aged people *see* older people
ageing 118–19, 138–9
  and gender 120
  and health 121–2
  population, Australia's 119–21
  population, cost of 122–4
Agency for Health Care and
  Policy and Research
  (AHCPR) 4, 13
alcohol 101, 102, 181
amphetamines 99, 102, 104
analgesia
  delivery and technology 9
  patient controlled 9

Anderson, Betty 42
asthma 182
Australian Health Ministers
  Advisory Council (AHMAC)
  188
Australian Institute of Health
  and Welfare (AIHW) 122
Australian Nursing Council
  (ANC) 15
Australian Wound Management
  Association 31, 32

Belize 43
Bland, Anthony 143–5, 155

Canada 43, 147, 167, 182
cancer
  and health care 181, 183
  pain and suffering 4, 7,
    12–13, 16
cannabis 100–1, 102, 104, 106
cardiovascular diseases 181,
  183
casemix 185–7, 198, 199
Charlesworth, Max 142, 155
charting 171–2

children and pain 10–11
Chile 43
chronic pain 11–12
clinical
  databases and references 170
  documentation 171
  pathways 170–1
Clinical Information Access
  Project (CIAP) 163–5, 174
Clinical Information Requirements
  Report 167
clinical information systems
  159–72, 174–5
  charting 171–2
  clinical databases and
    references 170
  clinical documentation 171
  clinical pathways 170–1
  discharge summary 169
  internet and modern health
    care 160, 161–5
  medical alerts 169
  order management 170
  patient acuity pathways 171
  patient history 170
  point-of-care systems 159,
    165–7, 174
  reporting 169–70
  results reporting 169–70
  status in Australia 167–8
  the technology 160, 165–7,
    168, 171–2, 174–5
cocaine 99, 102, 104–5
Coiera, Enrico 160
Consent to Medical Treatment
  and Palliative Care Act 1995
  (SA) 148
consumers and health care
  180–1, 184–5
coronary heart disease 182
Critical Care Information
  System 167

dementia 121–2
depressants 98, 99–100
detoxification 105, 111
Diers, Donna 53
discharge summary 169
diseases and health care 181
drug use 98, 115–17
  cost of 103–4
drug-related research 101–3
drugs
  dependence 104–5, 111
  depressants 99–100
  and detoxification 105, 111
  hallucinogens 100–1
  harm reduction strategies 107
  heroin trials 110–12
  illicit 103–4, 106–7
  injecting 100
  injecting rooms 109–10
  methadone maintenance
    treatment 106, 107–8, 111
  national strategy 101–3
  needle exchange programs
    105–6, 108–9
  prevention strategies 105–12
  primary interventions 105–6
  and prisons 102, 109
  secondary interventions 106
  stimulants 99
  supply and demand reduction
    106–7
  syringe exchange program
    105–6, 108–9
  tertiary interventions 106
  treatment 105–12
  types and their effects
    98–101
  withdrawal 104–5
Dying with Dignity: Interim
  Guidelines on Management
  146, 155

education, nurse practitioners
47–8
educational issues and pain 13–16
elderly people *see* older people
ethics and pain management
15–16
euthanasia 149–50, 151

Ford, Loretta 42

Germany 109, 110, 111
*Guide to Medical Informatics, the
Internet and Telemedicine, A*
160

hallucinogens 98, 100–1, 102
health and gender 120
health care
expenditure 179, 182, 187,
189, 193, 198
inefficiencies 183–4
as a market place 176–8, 184–7
and technology 181
health care system, Australian
187–9, 192–4
care delivery systems 188–9
casemix 185–7, 198, 199
financing 189
health practices 189
performance 182–4
pressures on 180–1
public 159, 178, 184
structure and scope 179–80,
189
health of older people *see* older
people
Henderson, Virginia 49
hepatitis 181
heroin 99–100, 102, 103, 104
trials 110–12
HIV 107
hospice movement 4, 13

illicit drugs and Australian
society 103–4, 106–7
injecting rooms 109–10
Inmate Health Survey 102
*Inquiry into Options for Dying
with Dignity* 148
institutional care and pain 6–8
International Association for the
Study of Pain (IASP) 5, 23
internet
and clinical information
systems 160, 161–5
and modern health care 162–5

life, extending 140–52, 155–6
defining terms 140–2
discontinuing treatment 147–9
and ending life 149–52
legislation 147–8, 149–51
and nurses 145–52, 155
patient resuscitation 146–7
placing a value on human
life 142–5
LSD 101

marijuana 100, 102, 106
medical alerts 169
Medical Benefits Scheme 179
medical profession 45–6, 69–70
Medical Treatment Act 1988
(Vic.) 148
*Medical Treatment (Enduring
Power of Attorney) Act 1990*
(Vic.) 148
Medicare 179–80, 182, 185
mental illness 181
and suicide 87–8, 95–6
methadone maintenance
treatment 106, 107–8, 111

naltrexone 111
National Drug Strategy 101–4

National Health and Medical
  Research Council (NH&MRC)
  6, 13, 14, 21, 22
National Health Survey 121, 122
Natural Death Act 1983 (SA) 147
Natural Death Act 1988 (NT) 148
needle exchange programs
  105–6, 108–9
neonatal pain 10
Netherlands 111, 151
New Aged Care Strategy 124
New Zealand 43–4
Nightingale, Florence 24, 30
NSW College of Nursing 54
NSW Nurse Practitioner
  Project 45, 49, 50, 53–4
  amendments to *Nurses Act
    1991* (NSW) 62
  amendments to *Poisons and
    Therapeutic Goods Act 1966*
    (NSW) 63
  authorisation of nurse
    practitioners 63–7
  framework for
    implementation 60–7
  legislative amendments 61
  and medical profession 46
  stage 1 46, 54
  stage 2 54–6
  stage 3 46, 47, 48, 56–60
NSW Nurses' Association 54
Nurse Practitioner Authorisation
  Committee 64, 65
nurse practitioners 40–2, 69–70
  and the aged 124–5, 127, 128
  Australia 44–50
  authorisation of 63–7
  clinical practice in Australia
    48–50, 66
  code of ethics 15
  education 47–8
  and extending life 145–52, 155

independence or autonomy
  46–7
international scene 42–4, 69
and pain management 15
politics 45–6
professional bodies 44
role of 42–4, 49, 59, 60, 69
rostering 195, 202–7
and wound management 31
see also NSW Nurse
  Practitioner Project
Nurses Act 1991 (NSW) 61, 62
*Nurses Amendment (Nurse
  Practitioners) Act 1988*
  (NSW) 61, 62
nursing issues and pain
  management 8–12
nursing resources
  analysis of staffing trends 211
  budget and staffing plan 198,
    216
  business planning model 195,
    196–202
  clinical and staffing profile
    212–13
  and clinical service
    requirements 199–202
  cost efficient 195
  key activity indicators 210
  master unit plan 214–15
  and rostering 202–7
  staffing details 199
  unit managed staffing (UMS)
    202–7
  unit managed staffing
    availability roster 217
  unit managed staffing hours
    accumulation and
    adjustment chart 218

older people
  and health 121–2

and pain 11
and relationship between
    nurses 128
Oncology Nursing Society of
    America 16
opium 98
order management 170

pain
  acute 14
  acute post-operative 9–10
  and aged care 4
  assessment, barriers related to
    5–6
  and cancer 4, 7, 12–13, 16
  in children 10–11
  chronic 11–12
  definition 5
  educational issues 13–16
  in the elderly 11
  measurement 6
  and models of care in
    institutions 6–8
  nature of 4–5
  neonatal 10
  procedural 8–9
  under treatment of 4
pain management 3, 21–3
  ethico-legal issues 15–16
  evidence-based practice
    14–15
  misuse of placebos 16–17
  and nurses 15
  and nursing issues 8–12
  and patients 6, 7, 8, 9, 14,
    15, 16–17
  practice guidelines 14–15
palliative care 4, 13, 150
patient
  acuity pathways 171
  history 170

and pain management 6, 7,
    8, 9, 14, 15, 16–17
  resuscitation 146–7
patient controlled analgesia
    (PCA) 9
Pharmaceutical Benefits
    Scheme (PBS) 179
placebos in pain management
    16–17
point-of-care systems 159,
    165–7, 174
Poisons and Therapeutic Goods
    Act 1966 (NSW) 61, 63
population
  Australia's ageing 119–21
  cost of ageing 122–4
post-operative pain 9–10
prisons and drugs 102, 109
procedural pain 8–9
Psychiatric Nurse Practitioner
    (PNP) 43
public health system 159

reporting, results 169–70
residential aged care 128–32
  acuity levels 131
  early hospital discharge 129–31
  multi-systems disorders 129
  relocation 131–2
results reporting 169–70
Rights of the Terminally Ill Act
    1995 (NT) 149
rostering 195, 202–7

Silver, Henry 42
smoking 101–2, 182
society, Australian
  and illicit drugs 103–4, 106–7
stimulants 98, 99
suicide 73–4, 90, 95–6
  assisted 149, 151
  attempted 84

comparison between states
    and other countries 78–9
cultural factors 80–3
defined 74–5
family dynamics 88–9
imitations 88
and mental illness 87–8, 95–6
methods used 80–3
prevalence 75–6
rates 76–9, 81, 84, 85, 89
risk factors 86–90
rural versus urban 85–6
socio-cultural factors 86–7
young people 76–8
Switzerland 110, 111
syringe exchange program
    105–6, 108–9

technology
    and analgesia delivery 9
    and clinical information
        systems 160, 165–7, 168,
        171–2, 174–5
    and health care 181
    see also internet
THC 101

tobacco 101–2
Torres Strait Islanders 183
tuberculosis 181

unit managed staffing (UMS)
    202–7
    availability roster 217
    hours accumulation and
        adjustment chart 218
United Kingdom 44, 69, 111,
    143, 146, 147, 150, 182
United States 42, 46, 50, 53,
    99, 107, 109, 130, 147, 161,
    167, 182

Wood Royal Commission 110
wound care 35
    cost of 32–5
wound management 24–6, 35,
    38–9
    and antiseptics 28
    challenging practice 26–9
    dressings 29–30
    and nurses 31–2
    specialisation 30–2
    tools of the trade 29–30

Printed in the United States
by Baker & Taylor Publisher Services